Nutrition for Sport

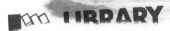

Nutrition
for Sport

Steve Wootton
Lecturer in Human Nutrition
Southampton University

Foreword by
Susan Campbell,
Director of the National Coaching Foundation,
Leeds

SPORTS PAGES
SIMON & SCHUSTER

A SPORTSPAGES BOOK

First published in paperback by
Simon & Schuster Ltd in 1989

Copyright © Steve Wootton, 1988
Reprinted 1990 (twice)

SPORTSPAGES
The Specialist Sports Bookshop
Caxton Walk
94-96 Charing Cross Road
London WC2H 0JG

Simon & Schuster Ltd
West Garden Place
Kendal Street
London W2 2AQ

Simon & Schuster of Australia Pty Ltd Sydney

British Library Cataloguing-in-Publication Data

Wootton Steve
Nutrition for sport: eating to improve performance.
1. Athletes—Nutrition. 2. Sports—Physiological aspects
1. Title
613.2'024796   TX. 361.A8

ISBN 0-671-69678-5 (*Paperback*)

Printed in Eras by DMD Ltd, Oxford
Printed and bound in Great Britain at
the University Press, Cambridge

Foreword

Dr Steve Wootton obtained his first degree in nutrition before working for his doctorate in exercise physiology under the guidance of Dr Clyde Williams at Loughborough University. Dr Wootton is now a lecturer in human nutrition at Southampton University. He is an acknowledged expert in sports nutrition and has a keen interest in all aspects of sport. Throughout his career Dr Wootton has been in constant touch with a range of practitioners and this has helped him to write a book which is highly relevant to everyone — performers, coaches, trainers, dietitians and sports nutritionists.

One of the outstanding features of the book is the way Dr Wootton has so clearly explained the theoretical principles underlying diet and performance. He has also linked this specialist knowledge with 'healthy eating' for living, so the book is valuable to everyone from the recreational player to the top flight sportsperson. Dr Wootton has explained how food is used by the body and provided advice on eating and diet for exercise. He has also stressed the importance of eating for training and the need for a sensible approach to preparation for competition. In so doing, he has exploded many of the myths about diet which are prevalent among performers.

Dr Wootton has evaluated the pros and cons of the high carbohydrate diet, the importance of fluid intake and how to approach weight control. Of special interest are his views on the intake of vitamins and minerals and his sensible approach to the use of supplements. At the end of the book there is a stimulating question and answer section and a most helpful glossary. Overall 'Nutrition for Sport' contains constructive advice on a new, sensible approach to diet for sport and is to be particularly recommended for the excellent way Dr Wootton applies theory to practice. It's got to be a 'must' for every person involved in sport.

Sue Campbell
Director
National Coaching Foundation

Acknowledgement

The thoughts expressed herein are not wholly original in that they represent the result of the collective views and opinions of many academics interested in nutrition, metabolism and exercise as well as many coaches and performers working throughout sport at all levels. It has been my great fortune to have been given the opportunity to work with, listen to and share thoughts with such committed and enthusiastic people — each striving to know more about how nutrition influences the way in which the body copes with the challenge of exercise. In particular I wish to express my thanks to: Prof Clyde Williams and Dr Adrianne Hardman (Loughborough University), Dr Ron Maughan (Aberdeen University Medical School), Prof Alan Jackson (Southampton University), Andy Etchells and Alison Turnbull (Running Magazine).

One final thought as this book goes to print is for Sally Jones who died so tragically during the final stages of editing the manuscript. Without her initial encouragement and persistence, this book would not have been started. This books is dedicated to the memory of Sally.

Contents

Preface

Over the last decade, it has been clearly acknowledged by government agencies, the food industry and the general public that good nutrition will have an impact on general health and well-being. Along with fitness, healthy eating has become the fashion of the 1980s. More recently, the competitive sportsman or woman has been made aware of the important role that nutrition can play in both training and competition for there is clear evidence to show that improved eating habits not only benefit health but also influence an individual's capacity to perform exercise. However, the new ideas have developed in a climate of considerable nutritional confusion and misinformation to the extent that many people have difficulty distinguishing myth from truth. Mistaken concepts have been used to support nutritional practices which are, at best, questionable and inadequate and, at worst, dangerous.

Nutrition is a relatively new science. In the past nutritionists were mainly associated with the prevention of nutritional disease or with animal husbandry but now the emphasis is on the promotion of health — so-called 'optimal nutrition'. Research in this area is progressing at a phenomenal rate; old beliefs are being superseded by new ideas, and beliefs of a decade ago are now turning out to be only partly correct or totally incorrect — such is scientific progress. Unfortunately the rate at which the new findings are disseminated to the general public is extremely slow. This may, in part, be due to a natural reluctance of many scientists to commit themselves to press without sufficient proof. Too often, sports nutritionists have been criticized for drawing too broad a conclusion on fact and for failing to support conclusions with sufficient evidence so perhaps their caution is understandable. It also has to be said that very few scientific studies have been performed using elite athletes and much of our understanding comes from laboratory studies (usually on male, physical education students) rather than out on the sports field; we know a considerable amount about the ways in which nutrition can alter performance during cycle ergometry but little about the applied aspects of sports nutrition. Care must be taken when applying observations to the vastly differing types of athletes, from young gymnasts to international shot-putters and Tour de France cyclists. The constraints placed upon us by lifestyle, likes and dislikes, coupled with an inherent biological variablility (so that no two individuals are identical) must be accommodated when applying dietary recommendations.

Others are less restrained and are quick to present their own interpretation of scientific research to the public. They may be neither in full possession of the facts nor understand fully the implications of the findings, but it often makes a good story and certainly sells books!

Many put forward their own personal dietary philosophies. They range from the self-styled 'experts' (successful performers or coaches who rely heavily on their own success to promote their ideas rather than on any direct evidence) to commercial organizations with a product to sell. The latter often depend in part on what can be called collective fadism to promote their products by using successful performers in their advertising campaigns. Many companies go to considerable lengths to suggest that their products will result in a marked and substantial improvement in performance — the inducements range from 10 per cent off a marathon time to the opportunity of becoming the world's greatest lover! Unfortunately such claims are totally without foundation and promotion relies heavily on the nutritional naivety of the consumer.

Finally all these factors interact against a backcloth of nutritional myth and custom that has been passed down through many generations of athletes. The athlete's continual quest for the 'winning edge' is absolute and leads to the adoption of many practices and beliefs which, while they may defy logic, are highly resistant to change.

With all these counter-influences, it is no wonder that there is confusion and misinformation in sports nutrition. However, these limitations should not prevent us from identifying those areas of nutrition where sufficient understanding does exist and translating the implications of this knowledge to the athlete. We know enough about the body's response to the challenge of exercise to be able to put forward sound principles, particularly in the area of energy metabolism and performance.

About the book

Athletes should be able to receive nutritional advice in much the same way that they expect sound training and medical advice. Those working closely with athletes, especially coaches and trainers, should have access to reliable nutritional information either by educating themselves in the sound principles or by taking the advice of professionally trained nutritionists and dietitians. But the responsibility does not lie just with the coach or trainer as athletes, with their own knowledge of nutrition, should be in a position to accept or reject the dietary advice offered to them: unfortunately this is the exception rather than the rule. The present degree of nutritional naivety, ignorance and confusion displayed by coaches and athletes alike only serves to further existing misunderstandings and, ultimately, to impair the development of individual athletes.

I hope this book will begin to set the record straight. Far from being just another guide to nutrition and healthy eating, the book explores the ways in which food can influence an athlete's ability to perform exercise. And, like most things, it is important to understand the basic principles of healthy eating first (Chaper 1) and then learn how to apply them in the sporting context. Interestingly and perhaps contrary to many athletes' beliefs, a successful sporting diet is not based on 'pills, powders and potions' (Chapter 9); there is no 'magic' solution to athletic success. The advice we can give to athletes about diet is the same as that being given to all members of the population so there need be no conflict between eating for performance and eating for health.

Chapters 2 and 3 are devoted to an explanation of how the food you eat is used to provide the energy necessary for muscular work. It is difficult to explain the relationship between food and exercise without a basic understanding of the principles of energy metabolism. Therefore, the book probably goes further than previous publications in describing the bio-chemical pathways of energy metabolism. Having grasped the underlying mechanism, you should be able to see how subtle alterations in nutrient intake can have profound effects on metabolism, which in turn will influence your ability to run, jump, swim and throw.

All exercise involves muscular work so the intricate structure and function of the different muscles is described in Chapter 4 as well as the factors that influence how the fuel (ie, food) for muscular work will be used, taking into account factors such as the type of exercise, the preceding diet and the duration of exercise.

All athletes experience fatigue during training and competition but there are ways to avoid it and enhance recovery following exercise, for example, refuelling with carbohydrates as soon after a training session as possible. The all-important topic of fluid is covered in Chapter 5, not only from the point of view of dehydration and rehydration but also body temperature regulation.

Later chapters deal with the controversial topic of carbo-loading, explaining the mechanism behind this technique and pointing out that not all athletes will benefit from it; sports that require athletes to lose or gain weight for competition; analysis of the pills, powders and potions presently on the market; the roles of vitamins and minerals.

The book finishes with a practical chapter on how both the performer and coach can implement the recommendations in the previous chapters and achieve an improvement in performance. As you will discover, you will have little success in improving your performance through diet unless you have grasped the concept of healthy eating. The final question-and-answer section illustrates a number of important concepts in practical sporting contexts.

It would be wrong to claim that changing your diet will automatically make you run faster or jump higher! Success lies in combining a sensible, healthy diet with training. Diet is one of many factors involved in improving athletic performance, but nonetheless a very important factor that is too often overlooked or abused.

Steve Wootton 1988

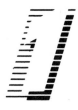

Nutrition: basic concepts

Nutritional terms explained

Nutrition The term nutrition describes the process by which materials from the environment are taken up by the body in order to provide the nutrients and energy necessary to keep the body alive and healthy.

Nutrients The food that you eat can be broken down into components called nutrients ie, carbohydrates, fats, proteins, alcohol, vitamins, minerals, trace elements, dietary fibre and water. Different foods are made of different proportions of nutrients. No one naturally occurring food contains sufficient amounts of each of these nutrients to meet the body's needs, hence the necessity to eat a wide variety of foods.

Diet Diets are best described as patterns of everyday eating habits and food selection which result in a specific nutrient consumption, for example, a low-fat diet, a weight-reducing diet, a high-fibre diet or a high-carbohydrate diet.

Digestion Digestion is the process by which the enzymes in your gut break down the larger compounds within foods to smaller compounds so that they may be absorbed by your body.

Absorption Absorption is the movement, in the stomach and small intestine, of digested food into the body tissues and blood. Not all of the food you eat is absorbed; this passes straight through your body and is eliminated as faeces.

Excretion Excretion is the removal of potentially noxious or poisonous end-products of metabolism from your body, normally in the urine and faeces.

Metabolism Metabolism is the sum of all chemical processes or reactions taking place in the body's organs and cells.

Energy

Energy is a difficult word to define as it has several accepted meanings in everyday life as well as a more precise scientific definition. To most people, energy can mean anything from atomic power stations to a man's

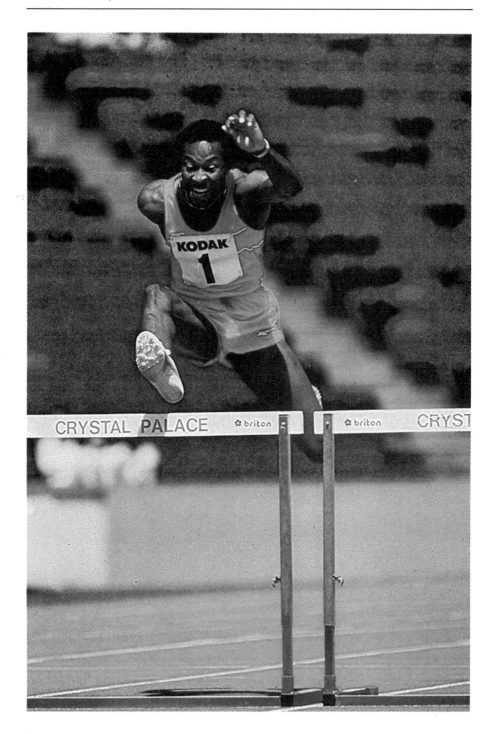

dynamism and *joie de vivre* and, in reality, the various common usages are quite compatible with the scientist's term: they all symbolize vigorous activity resulting in the ability to perform work. Obviously, you cannot induce a sense of *joie de vivre* simply by passing several thousand volts through your body. Yet it **is** important to realize that the feeling of a total lack of energy associated with overtraining can be influenced by altering the energy stores of the body!

In scientific terms, energy can be defined as the capacity to perform work. Although there are many different classifications of energy, such as chemical, thermal (or heat), mechanical, electrical, light and nuclear energy, they are all fundamentally the same and can be measured in the same units (see page 24).

The ultimate source of energy on earth is the sun. Energy radiated by the sun is harnessed by green plants as they synthesize complex organic substances (such as carbohydrates, proteins and fats) from simple inorganic materials (such as carbon dioxide and water) by a process called photosynthesis — literally, synthesis from sunlight. In the human body, all the energy is obtained from plant sources either directly by eating cereals, fruit and vegetables or indirectly by eating animal tissue (the animal gained energy in the first place by eating plants).

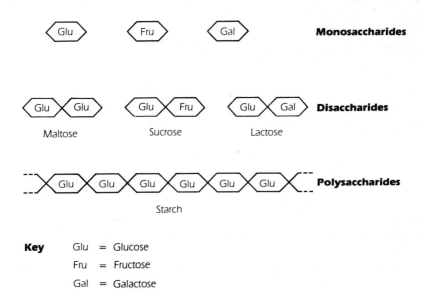

Key   Glu = Glucose
           Fru = Fructose
           Gal = Galactose

Fig.1.2. Schematic structure of the main forms of carbohydrate in food — monosaccharides, disaccharides and polysaccharides.

Carbohydrates

Carbohydrates are composed of carbon, hydrogen and oxygen. The basic unit of a carbohydrate is the monosaccharide; the most common monosaccharide in food is glucose. Glucose and other monosaccharides, such as fructose and galactose, are usually combined together in foods as larger compounds. When two monosaccharides are joined together they are termed a disaccharide. The most common disaccharide in the diet is sucrose or table sugar (one molecule of glucose combined with one molecule of fructose). Other disaccharides are maltose (two molecules of glucose — normally obtained when starch is broken down) and lactose (one glucose plus one galactose — the carbohydrate in milk).

Longer chains of monosaccharides, called polysaccharides, allow large quantities of glucose to be stored in the cells of plants (where the polysaccharide is starch) or animals (where it is in the form of glycogen). The process of digestion breaks the disaccharides and polysaccharides down to the basic monosaccharides which can then be absorbed by the body.

Whereas many of the different carbohydrates can be converted from one type to another within the body, the body has only a limited potential to produce glucose from substances other than carbohydrate (for example, it can produce glucose from proteins by a process called gluconeogenesis). So, to meet the body's requirements for carbohydrate, we must actually consume foods rich in carbohydrates.

Carbohydrates are important in maintaining the energy stores of the body (as glycogen) and are also used in the synthesis of important compounds in the body.

Complex carbohydrates and simple sugars

The best high-carbohydrate foods are those in which the carbohydrate exists in the natural unrefined state — the starchy foods containing complex carbohydrates (see table, page 9). The carbohydrate in these foods is mainly found in the form of polysaccharides that is, starch in whole grains and grain products. The best examples are the high-fibre foods, such as wholemeal or whole wheat bread, whole wheat pasta, cereals, pulses (peas and beans), vegetables and nuts. In addition to their starch content they also contain all the vitamins and minerals associated with the processes that metabolize the carbohydrate plus fibre.

The other high-carbohydrate foods are the sugary foods containing large amounts of refined or simple sugars. In these highly processed foods, the carbohydrates have been extracted from the natural source and broken down mainly into disaccharides and monosaccharides which can then be

Starchy carbohydrates	Simple sugars
Wholemeal bread flour and crispbreads	Sugars, syrups, jams, marmalades
Wholemeal pastas, brown rice	Confectionery: boiled sweets, chocolate
Pulses and legumes: peas, lentils, beans (kidney, haricot, baked beans etc,) pearl barley	toffee, fudge etc
	Sugary drinks: lemonade, cola, squashes, blackcurrant
Potatoes, sweetcorn, root vegetables	Drinking chocolate, malted bedtime
Cereals: Weetabix, Shredded Wheat, Branflakes, Puffed Wheat, porridge, sugar-free muesli	drinks
	Sugar-coated cereals, sugary cakes, biscuits, pastries, fruit pies and
Nuts: peanuts (unsalted), brazils, hazelnuts, chestnuts, almonds, etc	crumbles, jellies, cheesecake, ice cream, fruit yoghurt, tinned fruit in
Fresh fruit: apples, pears, oranges, bananas, grapes	syrup, sweet custard, milk puddings, sweet pickles
Dried fruit: currants, sultanas, apricots, prunes etc	
Tinned fruit in natural juice	

Table 1.1 Foods rich in carbohydrates.

rapidly absorbed following relatively little digestion. Examples include sweet foods, such as sugar, preserves and confectionery. While they contain carbohydrate, they usually contain little in the way of vitamins, minerals, trace elements and fibre, but often a lot of fat. So they are considered to be less nutritious than starchy carbohydrate foods rich in fibre.

Fats

Fat's basic component is the triglyceride which consists of a glycerol base with three fatty acids attached. The difference between the various types of fats depends upon which fatty acids are in the triglyceride. Fatty acids are chains of carbon atoms (usually 16–20 carbon atoms long) which can either be saturated with hydrogen atoms (the saturated fatty acids normally found in animal fats) or contain relatively fewer hydrogen atoms (the unsaturated or polyunsaturated fatty acids commonly found in vegetable fats and oils). Two of these unsaturated fatty acids (linoleic and linolenic acid) must be eaten in the diet and are thus called essential fatty acids. Cholesterol is not a fatty acid, but a type of fat found mainly in animal produce, for example, egg yolks.

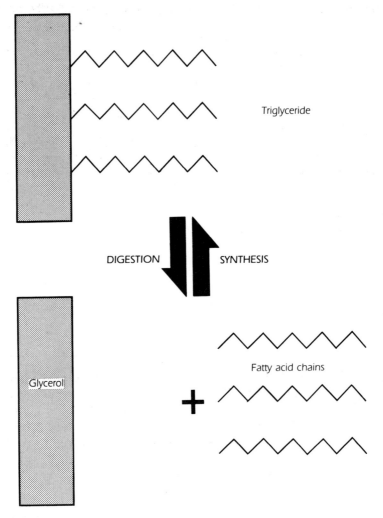

Triglyceride

DIGESTION   SYNTHESIS

Fatty acid chains

Glycerol

+

Fig.1.3 Schematic structure of a triglyceride (fat) comprising glycerol and three fatty acid chains.

When digested, triglycerides are broken down into fatty acids and glycerol, which can then be absorbed. Fats are important nutrients, not only as a source of energy, but also to synthesize many important compounds and tissues vital for the normal functioning of the body. Even so, it is generally believed that we eat far too much fat in our diet, particularly the saturated fats. (For more information on the associated risk of coronary heart disease, see page 18.)

Visible fats	Hidden fats	Low-fat alternatives
Butter, margarine, lard, suet, dripping	Meat, especially beef, pork, lamb, bacon, ham, duck	Skimmed milk; skimmed milk products; low fat cheeses, e.g. cottage,
Oils (vegetable, fish, etc)	Oily fish, e.g. mackerel, sardines, pilchards, salmon, herrings	curd, low fat spreads; use natural yoghurt instead of cream.
Fatty meat, pork crackling and scratchings		
Skin on chicken and duck	Meat pies, and pasties, sausages, burgers, pâtés, salami, pork pies etc.	White meats — poultry (remove the skin); white fish, e.g. plaice, cod, coley, sole, shellfish; crustaceans, e.g. crab.
	Cheese (except curd, cottage and low fat types)	
	Whole milk, cream, creamy puddings, cheesecakes	
	Nuts, olives, avocado pears	
	Chips, crisps, fried foods	
	Mayonnaise, peanut butter	

Table 1.2 Foods rich in fat, both visible and hidden fat, with suggestions for low-fat alternatives.

Proteins

Proteins are large molecules which, when broken down in the gut, yield simple units called amino acids: molecules containing carbon, hydrogen, oxygen and nitrogen (some also contain sulphur). There are twenty-one amino acids and, just as the twenty-six letters of the alphabet can be combined into thousands of different words, the amino acids can combine together to create a vast number of peptides and proteins required by the body. Some amino acids are interchangeable with others, but there are at least eight amino acids which the body cannot make for itself. These are termed the essential amino acids and they must be eaten in the diet. It is not protein itself that your body needs, but a sufficient quantity of each of the amino acids.

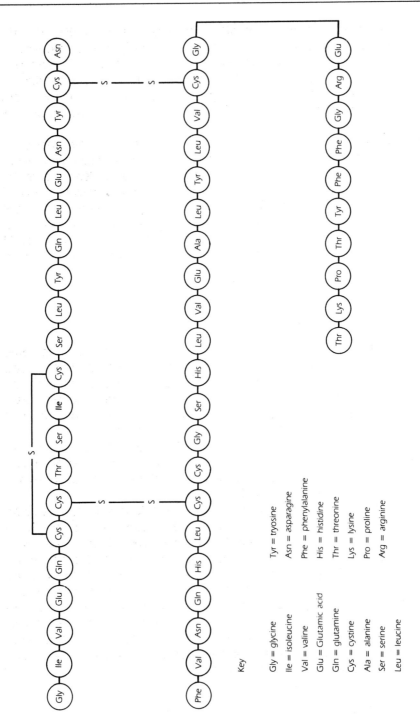

Key

Gly = glycine
Ile = isoleucine
Val = valine
Glu = Glutamic acid
Gln = glutamine
Cys = cystine
Ala = alanine
Ser = serine
Leu = leucine

Tyr = tryosine
Asn = asparagine
Phe = phenylalanine
His = histidine
Thr = threonine
Lys = lysine
Pro = proline
Arg = arginine

Fig.1.4 Schematic structure of human insulin as an example of a protein comprising a specific sequence of amino acids.

Amino acids are required primarily to manufacture the structural components of many tissues (for example, muscle) haemoglobin, hormones and digestive enzymes. They are continually being formed into proteins and then broken down again into amino acids as required. Under extreme conditions, such as starvation and when relatively little energy can be derived from depleted fat and carbohydrate reserves, amino acids may be used to provide energy.

When you eat more protein than you need, the excess amino acids are broken down, the nitrogen excreted and the rest of the molecule used to produce energy, either immediately or after storage. Protein deficiency in the athlete is rare, in fact we generally consume too much — particularly animal protein. There is little evidence to suggest that you need to greatly increase your normal protein intake even during very heavy training — the increase in requirement is probably very small. However, during growth spurts in childhood and adolescence, a relatively larger amount of protein is needed in the diet.

Animal and vegetable proteins

High amounts of essential amino acids are found in meat, fish and some dairy produce, but the contribution that can be made by non-animal sources, such as cereals, pulses and nuts should not be underestimated. The traditional view of 'first class'/complete (or animal) and 'second class'/incomplete (or vegetable) proteins tends to devalue vegetable protein as of little nutritional value; it stems from the observation that the protein found in plants is of inferior biological quality compared with animal proteins, such as those found in eggs and milk. While vegetable proteins contain lower amounts of **some** of the essential amino acids than are found in animal proteins, they are far from lacking in amino acids.

In addition, the biological quality of any vegetable protein can easily be improved by eating a wide variety of vegetables, grains and nuts (see Table 1.3). Combining a vegetable protein low in one essential amino acid with another high in that amino acid, so that they complement each other, results in a more balanced supply of amino acids. For example, cereals are generally high in two particular amino acids, methionine and tryptophan, yet low in lysine. On the other hand, pulses tend to contain relatively high amounts of lysine yet little methionine and tryptophan. A combination of the two results in a protein food complete with sufficient quantities of all three amino acids. It is surprising how man's palate naturally combines such foods — baked beans or peanut butter on toast, for example.

Animal sources	**Vegetable sources**
(Tend to be high in fat)	(High in carbohydrate and fibre)
Meat, poultry, offal	Legumes, lentils, peas
Fish, shellfish	Beans, e.g. haricot, mung, butter beans,
Milk, cheese, yoghurt	baked beans
Eggs	Nuts and seeds
	Bread, potatoes, cereals, pasta, rice, etc

Table 1.3 Foods rich in proteins.

Vitamins

Vitamins are chemical compounds needed in minute amounts to perform specific bodily functions — yet they are either not made by the body or only in insufficient amounts.

As the vitamins were discovered, they were labelled first with letters then, once identified, given a specific name, for example, vitamin A became retinol, vitamin B_1 became thiamine, etc. Now they are broadly classified into those which can be dissolved in organic solvents (the fat-soluble vitamins: A, D, E, and K) and those which can be dissolved in water (the water-soluble vitamins: the B group and C).

In Western countries obvious signs of a specific vitamin deficiency are rare in either the general public or in sportspeople. However, the possibility that low vitamin levels in the body may impair performance cannot be overlooked.

The intake of any particular nutrient will obviously be related to the volume of food eaten. If the total energy intake decreases (for example, with repeated episodes of energy restriction), it may be difficult to consume sufficient vitamins and minerals unless specific foods are eaten which are high in vitamins and minerals while being low in energy. Thus care should be taken to avoid hyponutrition (inadequate food intake).

While overconsumption of vitamins and minerals from food is very rare, it is easy to consume 10–100 times more than is required by using concentrated vitamins and mineral supplements. Care should be taken as the body cannot cope with non-physiological (abnormally high) intakes of many vitamins without serious side-effects. Vitamin toxicity has been noted specifically with vitamins A, D, E and K (the fat-soluble vitamins). It should also be noted that pangamic acid (the so-called vitamin B_{15}) is not really a vitamin, and there is strong evidence that certain forms of B_{15} may be harmful to health.

For more detailed information on vitamins, see Chapter 8.

Minerals, electrolytes and trace elements

Minerals are chemicals required by the body in very small amounts, and include iron, sodium, potassium, calcium, phosphorus and magnesium. Generally they exist as mineral salts (such as sodium chloride — table salt) but, when dissolved in water, they break down to their constituent elements (in this case sodium and chloride ions). In this state they are commonly called electrolytes.

Other chemicals, called trace elements, are required in even smaller amounts, and include copper, zinc and fluoride. All essential for life, they are important components of bone, connective tissue, haemoglobin, hormones and many enzymes within the body. However, as with vitamins, excess consumption of certain minerals (iron, for example), particularly as supplements, can result in an excessive accumulation that may be damaging. For more detailed information on minerals and trace elements, see Chapter 8.

Fibre

As dietary fibre is not actually absorbed by the body it is often ignored as an important part of the diet. Fibre is the non-digestible carbohydrate material that forms the skeleton of plants and is also found on the outside of seeds, peas, beans and vegetables. So when outer layers of food are removed by milling (as with flour) or by peeling, much of the all-important fibre is discarded.

Fibre provides non-energy-containing bulk to food as it passes through the body. It is essential to the proper functioning of the gut: insufficient fibre in the diet has been related to many Western diseases (such as constipation, gallstones, etc).

Water

Water is one of the most important nutrients required by the body and performs many vital functions. It is the body's main transportation mechanism, conveying nutrients, waste metabolites and internal secretions (for example, hormones) to target tissues. Water constitutes the prime component of many cells and, as it is a powerful ionizing agent, it controls the distribution of numerous electrolytes within cells and throughout the body. Similarly, oxygen and carbon dioxide, as well as hydrogen ions which affect acidity changes, are dissolved in water.

Of prime importance is the role water plays in temperature regulation, particularly during exercise (Chaper 5). Cellular water absorbs the heat generated during energy liberation in the cell and transports it to the skin to be dispersed into the environment. The excretion of sweat (which is mainly water) provides the capacity for evaporative heat loss with the resultant cooling effect on the body. It should be noted that even small losses of water (2–3 per cent loss of body weight) can seriously impair performance.

Alcohol

Alcohol (the product of the fermentation of carbohydrate by yeasts) may make a major contribution to a person's total energy intake. However, it differs from carbohydrate and fat in that it cannot be used by muscle to provide energy during exercise. Also, it cannot be used to provide a rapid release of energy on demand because it is metabolized slowly by the liver at a constant rate. So any energy derived from alcohol in excess of energy requirements would simply be stored as body fat or used by the liver to provide energy. Remember also that excessive alcohol consumption can cause serious damage to the liver.

Healthy eating

Ill-health is one of the most important factors limiting the quality of life but it is very difficult to find out precisely what determines good health free from major illness. Certainly there is no one simple and clear way to guarantee it: many different elements are involved.

By studying both genetic and environmental factors it is possible to predict which physical characteristics parents will pass on to their children, and to find out whether a child will be more or less predisposed to a major illness or disease (such as haemophilia or cystic fibrosis) afflicting one or both parents or a blood relative. Yet our genetic makeup cannot be altered. In contrast, the environment we create for ourselves can be modified to a certain extent. Smoking, exercise, the type of food we eat and the manner in which we cause and cope with the stresses of everyday life, are all amenable to change. Athletes, along with the rest of the population, should consider these points. Athletes are not immune from illnesses such as heart disease just because they exercise. Fortunately, the types of foods you should eat to improve sporting performance are identical to those that are best for health — so there is no conflict!

What is the healthiest diet?

As it is both impractical and often unethical to carry out longterm feeding studies on humans, much of our understanding about the healthiest type of food and the relative balance of nutrients comes from examining the incidence of disease in populations with very different eating habits and diets — so called epidemiological studies. Such evidence must be interpreted cautiously as there are genetic differences between populations and diet is only one aspect of lifestyle that may determine health. Nevertheless, general trends can be identified and are often called risk factors — one of these is diet. The greater the number of risk factors, the greater the chance of developing a particular disease.

One of the major differences observed between populations with and without a high incidence of longterm disease (such as obesity, heart disease and gut-related disorders) is the level of fat intake in the diet. For example, in countries where the incidence of coronary heart disease is low, the majority of energy in the diet comes from carbohydrate sources — and mainly in the form of starchy foods rich in complex carbohydrates rather than refined sugars. Not only does this form of carbohydrate contain the most vitamins and minerals, but also a high level of dietary fibre.

Additional evidence may also be derived from what are termed intervention studies (for example, examining the changes in the incidence of coronary heart disease after altering the type of fat in the diet). Such studies take time, however, and it is very difficult to change one factor without affecting others. While the consequences of longterm dietary changes have yet to be evaluated, such modifications in eating habits have been put into practice in the short term with mixed results.

Dietary guidelines

A consensus of opinion on diet and health is emerging among expert medical groups that advocates certain dietary changes for the general population. Around twenty years ago, a set of recommendations for healthy eating was published in the USA. Since then, most Western countries have promoted similar goals or guidelines in an attempt to prevent or postpone the development of major diseases, from obesity and tooth decay to coronary heart disease, certain cancers, strokes and diabetes (see Appendix III on page 178).

These dietary recommendations are not just for those who have shown signs of these diseases but for the population as a whole. To summarize the main points, the population should:

- control energy intake
- eat less fat, particularly saturated fat
- eat more starchy foods rich in fibre
- eat less refined and processed sugars
- eat less salt
- drink less alcohol.

Body weight

The amount of energy you consume should be defined in terms of those appropriate for the maintenance of an optimal body weight with adequate exercise; those people doing more than adequate exercise will need a higher energy intake. These optimal body weights should be appropriate for height and sex (see Figure 1.5). No increase in body weight should be allowed for once adulthood is reached, so any 'middle-age spread' is unacceptable. People should be encouraged to adjust their diet and to take more exercise so that adult body weight is kept within the optimum limits throughout life.

Even a moderate degree of overweight is important in health terms and should not be overlooked. Risks associated with excess weight are not confined to those who are substantially obese because there is a progressive rise in illness and death rates with even small increases in weight. Mild degrees of excess weight are particularly important in those with a family pattern of coronary heart disease or diabetes as well as those who already have high blood pressure.

Dietary fat

Many professional and governmental committees, both nationally and internationally, have reviewed the evidence relating to the causes of coronary heart disease (CHD). There is now a strong consensus of opinion that CHD can be reduced by cutting the amount of fat in the diet to about 30 per cent of the total energy intake, specifically reducing the consumption of saturated fats to less than 10 per cent. A typical daily fat intake for a man in a Western country at the moment is around 100–150 g/4–5 oz and around 75–130 g/3–5 oz for a woman. This provides about 40–45 per cent of the total energy in the diet. By cutting the fat content of our diet to no more than 30 per cent of the total daily energy intake, this would mean that men should

18

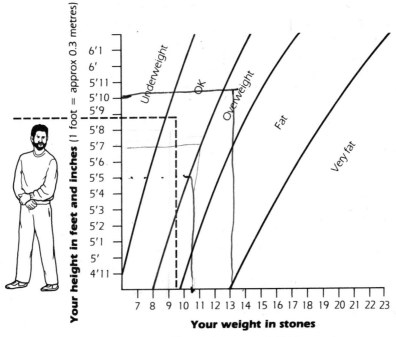

Your height in feet and inches (1 foot = approx 0.3 metres)

Your weight in stones

(1 pound = approx 0.45 kilograms)

Underweight Maybe you need to eat a bit more, but go for well-balanced nutritious foods and don't just fill up on fatty and sugary foods. If you are very underweight, see your doctor about it.

OK You're eating the right **quantity** of food but you need to be sure that you are getting a healthy **balance** in your diet.

Overweight You should try to lose weight.

Fat You need to lose weight

Very fat You need to lose weight. You would do well to see your doctor who might be able to refer you to a dietitian.

Fig.1.5 Are you a healthy weight? To find out, take a straight line across from your height (without shoes) and a line up from your weight (without clothes). Put a mark where the two lines meet. (Remember that the categories on the chart take no account of body composition so the muscular but lean athlete may appear overweight for his height.) The chart should only be used as a general guide. If you feel that you need to lose weight, aim to lose 1–2 lb/week until you get down to the 'OK' range. Go for fibre-rich foods and cut down on fat, sugar and alcohol. You will need to take extra exercise.

19

not exceed 75–125 g/3–5 oz of fat and women, 50–100 g/2–4 oz.

Controlled dietary experiments have shown that a high saturated fat diet tends to push up the level of fatty substances in the blood, in particular cholesterol, and this affects some people more than others; the extent appears to depend on hereditary factors. Similarly people with a high blood cholesterol level are more likely to suffer a heart attack or angina.

Cholesterol in the diet was itself originally believed to be the principal cause of high blood cholesterol levels, but more recent evidence suggests that blood cholesterol levels are not always related to the dietary intake of cholesterol; simply cutting out cholesterol from the diet will not always lower blood cholesterol levels. This is because not all of the body's cholesterol comes from food. It is made naturally within the body and, as an important component of cellular membranes, it is vital for the essential functioning of our cells. We make as much cholesterol as we need and, as we take in a certain amount of cholesterol in our food (from animal produce), we make automatic adjustments in synthesis and removal to compensate for changes in dietary intake. In this way the level of cholesterol in our bodies, and blood in particular, should remain relatively constant. This balance can be upset by:

● Eating too much fat, saturated fats in particular
● Eating too much cholesterol so that our compensating mechanisms cannot cope or
● Having an inbuilt fault in the compensating system so that the control of cholesterol synthesis and clearance is impaired.

It pays to aim to eat less saturated fat and cholesterol — this means consuming less fat in general and less animal fats in particular.

Carbohydrate and fibre intake

It is recommended that, in general, we cut our sugar intake by half. Although you may be using less sugar as sucrose, you may still be eating other sugars used in manufactured foods. Along with reducing fat intake, a reduction in sugar intake will lower the total energy content of the diet. Energy intakes should be maintained by replacing foods rich in fat and sugar with low-fat foods, the energy coming mainly from unprocessed food sources, such as bread (preferably whole grain), potatoes, fruit and other vegetables — each increasing by 25–30 per cent. Such changes will also have the desirable effect of increasing total dietary fibre intake.

A typical daily carbohydrate intake for a man in a Western country would be around 250–400 g/9–14 oz per day, for a woman around 150–300 g/ 5–11 oz. This would provide approximately 40–45 per cent of the total energy in a person's diet. The latest recommendations for healthy eating suggest that we should try to eat more carbohydrate so that it provides about half or possibly more of the energy in our daily diet.

A typical daily fibre intake would be around 10–20 g/½–¾ oz for both men and women. The latest recommendation is that you should increase your fibre intake to about 30 g/1½ oz per day by eating foods naturally high in fibre. You should bear in mind that the excessive consumption of bran (a popular source of fibre) can have unfortunate side-effects, such as impaired mineral absorption or mechanical obstruction of the gut.

Protein intake

A typical daily protein intake for a man in a Western country would be around 100 g/4 oz and around 75 g/3 oz for a woman. This would provide approximately 10–15 per cent of the total energy intake. While this is in accordance with the total protein intake in the latest recommendations, care should be taken to avoid excessive consumption of animal proteins (particularly red meat and processed meat products) because of their high saturated fat content. A greater proportion of protein should come from vegetable sources.

Salt

It is recommended that excessive salt intakes be reduced, as high salt consumption is associated with high blood pressure. It is believed that excess salt early in life can even set the stage for later development of high blood pressure. Therefore the recommendation to reduce salt is intended for everyone, not just the hypertensive. It is not possible to determine in advance which of us will be susceptible to the effects of salt.

Alcohol

Attention should also be given to the overall alcohol intake. We do not usually think of alcohol as 'food' but it does contribute a significant number of calories (see page 152).

A balanced diet

The idea of a 'balanced' diet stems from the recognition that an appropriate mixture of foods is necessary to provide the body with minimum amounts of nutrients. These needs are less likely to be met if the diet contains only a small variety of foods. By ensuring that several different foods are consumed, one item rich in a particular nutrient will 'balance' the lack of this nutrient in another food. An alternative approach is to think of a healthy diet as a 'varied' diet. However the introduction of a great variety of food alone is unlikely to alter disease patterns.

Recommended intakes of nutrients

Although it is very difficult to say how much you should eat of any one nutrient each day, governments have issued tables (see Appendix III page 178) of recommended intakes for certain nutrients.

The recommended intake or allowance of a nutrient each day is defined as the amount sufficient or more than sufficient to cover the nutritional needs of practically all persons in a **population**: this does not take into account additional nutritional needs arising from illness, such as infections, disorders of the gastrointestinal tract or metabolic abnormalities. The intake of one nutrient is based on the assumption that the requirements for energy and all other nutrients are being fully met at the same time. There is no evidence to suggest that intakes greatly in excess of the recommended amounts are of any benefit; indeed, excess intakes of energy and certain nutrients (for example, fat soluble vitamins) may even be harmful. In addition, it has not been proved that exercise influences your requirements for specific nutrients.

Although the values are listed on a daily basis, it does not mean that each must be met in full every day. Your body has the capacity to store any nutrient in sufficient quantity to last at least a few days and it can therefore cope with irregular intakes to some degree. The recommended intakes must take into account many factors, including age, size, growth rate and level of activity. Bear in mind that the allowances should only be used as a useful benchmark or minimum target intake against which actual nutrient intakes can be compared.

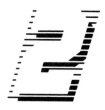

From food
to energy

It is possible to calculate that, in general terms, a typical daily energy intake for a man in a westernized country is between 4.2 MJ/1000 kcal and 20.8 MJ/5000 kcal, and for a woman it is between 4.2 MJ/1000 kcal and 14.7 MJ/3500 kcal. But it would be wrong, and possibly dangerous, to generalize further and say that a particular type of sportsperson, such as a footballer, needs a certain amount of energy each day; this amount is dependent on factors specific to individual footballers (eg, size, shape, degree of exercise) not footballers in general. For the same reasons, a table of energy expenditures for different sports (eg, 15 minutes of gymnastics expends 420 kJ/100 kcal of energy) can be very misleading — athletes of various shapes and sizes within a sport will exercise at different speeds within a given time limit and therefore will expend vastly different amounts of energy.

By the end of this chapter, you will have a better idea of energy measurement and metabolism but for the time being you should bear in mind the following:

- If you consume more energy than you actually require, the majority of the excess will be stored as fat and your weight will increase.
- If you eat an insufficient amount of energy, you will need to call upon your body's energy stores to meet the demand for energy and you will lose weight.

Energy metabolism

Living cells transform the potential chemical energy available within food into other forms of energy for normal bodily functions — mechanical energy for movement, thermal energy for keeping warm, electrical energy for conduction of a signal along a nerve, and, in some organisms, light. The sum total of these processes by which energy is transformed and utilized in the living organism is called metabolism.

The nutritional problems arising in energy metabolism involve the balancing of energy intake against energy expenditure. Potential energy is stored in food by being 'trapped' in the chemical bonds within the molecules of carbohydrate, protein and fat as they are being synthesized. By a series of processes whereby food is consumed, digested, absorbed and then assimilated into storage forms of protein, carbohydrate and fat within the body, this energy can be made available as it is needed for the physiological processes requiring energy.

Energy is not just required for muscular work, as in exercise. A huge variety of physiological processes cannot take place without energy, for example, the synthesis of proteins, fats and carbohydrates and the conduction of electrical impulses along the nerve. In fact, nearly every process within cells requires energy in one form or another. As energy is needed, it can be made available by breaking the chemical bonds in which it is 'trapped' so that the desired process may take place. Without the continual supply of energy, cells could not function properly.

How is energy measured?

In order to work out how energy intake and expenditure are balanced by the body, we must be able to measure energy accurately. All processes of energy metabolism ultimately depend on the complete combustion of foodstuff, in the presence of oxygen within the cell, in order to liberate the potential energy stored within the food. This process — called oxidation — results in the liberation of energy, with carbon dioxide and water. Part of the energy can be harnessed in a convenient form of energy currency, adenosine triphosphate (ATP) (see page 34) to permit the physiological or metabolic process to take place. The remainder is given off as heat. When energy is required by the cell, ATP is broken down and the energy which has been temporarily stored within the high-energy bonds of ATP is released.

Units of energy

All energy transformations ultimately result in the production of heat as a waste product. This is why the most commonly used unit of energy is the calorie and the measurement of energy expenditure is called calorimetry. Simply defined, a calorie is the heat required to raise 1 g of water by 1°C but, since the calorie is a very small quantity, the kilocalorie is more frequently used (1 kcal = 1000 calories).

A newer system for measuring energy units called joules (J), kilojoules (kJ) and megajoules (MJ). A joule is a more accurate way of defining energy and is appropriate to use for all its different forms; a joule is the energy expended when 1 kilogram is moved 1 metre by a force of 1 newton. It is simple to make an approximate conversion from kilocalories to kilojoules:

1 kcal = 4.2 kJ;

1 MJ = 1000 kJ = 240 kcals.

Measuring the energy content of food

In order to measure the energy content of a given food, a technique called bomb calorimetry is commonly employed. The food stuff is placed in a small chamber (the 'bomb'), exposed to a high pressure of oxygen (in the presence of a platinum catalyst), and ignited by a small electrical current. All the organic material is combusted completely and the heat liberated is measured.

In the body, the situation is slightly different, however, because not all the energy within food is completely combusted or absorbed. The amount of energy liberated within the body after full oxidation varies considerably

Foodstuff	Heat of combustion when fully combusted kJ/g (kcal/g)	Percentage of energy ultimately available %	Conversion factor used to calculate energy yield kJ/g (kcal/g)
Carbohydrate			
Starch	17.2 (4.12) ⎫	99	16 (3.75)
Glucose	15.5 (3.69) ⎭		
Fats			
Butter	38.2 (9.12)	95	37 (9)
Proteins			
Meat	22.4 (5.35) ⎫	92	17 (4)
Egg	23.4 (5.58) ⎭		
Alcohol	29.7 (7.10)	100	29 (7)

Table 2.1 The heat of combustion, available energy and conversion factor for carbohydrates, fats, proteins and alcohol. Note that fat yield approximately twice as much energy as carbohydrates and proteins so should be eaten in moderation.

25

between different types of food. For example, 1 g of fat yields more than twice as much energy as 1 g of carbohydrate — 37 kJ/9 kcal compared with 16 kJ/4 kcal. Proteins yield 16 kJ/4 kcal per gram while alcohol yields 29 kJ/7 kcal per gram.

Measuring the rate of energy metabolism

The rate of energy metabolism in man can be measured in several ways. As all metabolic processes ultimately involve oxidation and result in heat production, there are two principal methods of measuring energy expenditure: directly, by measuring the heat given off by the body; and indirectly, by measuring the rate at which oxygen is consumed (see fig. 2.3, page 35).

At rest, most of the energy resulting from all the transformations necessary to maintain man's life processes is in the form of heat. Apart from providing the energy to support bodily functions, this also serves to control the temperature of the body so that these processes can function optimally. Even during exercise, when an increasing proportion of energy is used to generate mechanical work, some 75–80 per cent is still released as heat because of the relative inefficiency of man as a machine.

Measuring heat production is the most appropriate way of assessing energy expenditure, but in practice it does have several drawbacks. Fortunately, the rate of oxygen consumption — that is, the rate at which oxygen is taken up by the subject and retained within the body through respiration — is directly related to heat production. So measuring the rate of oxygen consumption provides a good estimate of the metabolic rate. In the process of oxidizing the molecules of carbohydrate, fat and protein within the cell, oxygen is used and carbon dioxide is given off, in relative amounts which depend upon the mixture of fuels being combusted. So by measuring oxygen uptake and carbon dioxide production, it is possible to determine what fuels are being combusted by the tissues as well as measure the rate of energy expenditure.

Oxygen uptake

Normally the rate of oxygen uptake is determined by collecting the expired air from an individual, either at rest or during exercise, and measuring both the amount of oxygen removed from the atmosphere and carbon dioxide produced. The oxygen uptake ($\dot{V}O_2$) of an individual at rest is relatively low — around 0.2–0.4 litres per minute. As an individual starts to perform exercise, the rate at which energy is required increases, and so does the rate of energy metabolism and the rate of oxidation. This is reflected in the increase in $\dot{V}O_2$ by the body as a whole. Oxygen uptake continues to increase with the exercise intensity until a point is reached where it does not increase further despite the individual being able to work at still higher intensities (see Figure 2.1). The highest $\dot{V}O_2$ achieved is called the maximal oxygen uptake ($\dot{V}O_2$max) and is an expression of the individual's maximal physiological capacity for the transport and utilization of oxygen. The individual's $\dot{V}O_2$max is determined primarily by hereditary factors although it may be influenced to some extent (around 5–15 per cent) by training or the lack of it. The greatest $\dot{V}O_2$max is generally seen in the elite endurance athlete — particularly rowers, cyclists and marathon runners — and values as high as 5–6 litres per minute have been recorded. A typical $\dot{V}O_2$max for an untrained individual is around 2–3 litres per minute.

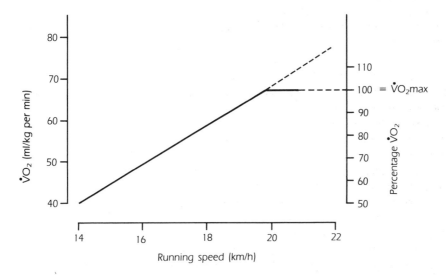

Fig.2.1 The relationship between the oxygen cost ($\dot{V}O_2$) of running at various speeds (with running speeds expressed as a percentage of $\dot{V}O_2$max). Once an athlete has achieved 100 per cent $\dot{V}O_2$max, he will be still able to increase his running speed significantly.

Relative exercise intensity

If two people run at the same speed and use the same amount of oxygen they do not always experience the same degree of physiological and metabolic stress. One runner may find the exercise particularly challenging, while the other is working comfortably, which may in part be explained by differences in their $\dot{V}O_2$max. If, on the other hand, the oxygen uptake at a given exercise intensity is expressed as a percentage of the individual's $\dot{V}O_2$max, it is possible to set an exercise intensity such that both runners are working at similar degrees of stress. If both individuals work at the same relative exercise intensity (as a percentage of $\dot{V}O_2$max), then the cardio-vascular, thermoregulatory and (to some degree) the metabolic responses to the task will be comparable. This concept of 'relative exercise intensity' makes it possible to compare the way in which the body responds to the challenge of exercise in individuals of differing ability and training status.

Most endurance sports take place at exercise intensities of 60–90 per cent $\dot{V}O_2$max. Many sports involve intensities considerably greater than $\dot{V}O_2$max; for example, in sprinting the rate at which energy is used is two to four times greater than that observed at $\dot{V}O_2$max.

How is energy released from food and stored in the body?

In nature, energy is stored within cells primarily in chemical bonds of the storage forms of both carbohydrate (as glycogen) and fat (as triglyceride); these are more energetically compact and efficient than the basic components, monosaccharides and fatty acids. Amino acids and proteins are not usually held in a storage form as such, but generally play a functional role as proteins and peptides which can be broken back down to amino acids as required.

As the human body cannot absorb starch or glycogen and triglyceride directly, they must first be broken down into the basic components by the process of digestion before entering the body tissues. Once the metabolic fate of these basic components has been determined by the body, they may be used in the basic form as required or recombined back into the storage forms until needed. It should be remembered that the human body does not store carbohydrate in any appreciable amount other than as glucose in glycogen. As the liver can convert most forms of carbohydrate from one form to another, it is not necessary to store every different type of carbohydrate.

'Turnover' — fine-tuning the energy supply

The process of digestion and the primary sites of absorption of nutrients are summarized in Figure 2.2. The digestion, absorption, assimilation and utilization of nutrients to provide us with energy must be tightly controlled. The body must be able to recognize when nutrients are entering the system (for example, after eating a meal) so that the appropriate metabolic response — the synthesis or storage of the nutrients — is initiated. The concentration

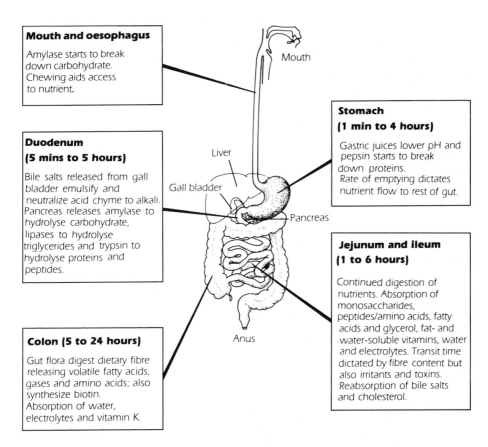

Mouth and oesophagus

Amylase starts to break down carbohydrate. Chewing aids access to nutrient.

Duodenum

(5 mins to 5 hours)

Bile salts released from gall bladder emulsify and neutralize acid chyme to alkali. Pancreas releases amylase to hydrolyse carbohydrate, lipases to hydrolyse triglycerides and trypsin to hydrolyse proteins and peptides.

Stomach

(1 min to 4 hours)

Gastric juices lower pH and pepsin starts to break down proteins. Rate of emptying dictates nutrient flow to rest of gut.

Jejunum and ileum

(1 to 6 hours)

Continued digestion of nutrients. Absorption of monosaccharides, peptides/amino acids, fatty acids and glycerol, fat- and water-soluble vitamins, water and electrolytes. Transit time dictated by fibre content but also irritants and toxins. Reabsorption of bile salts and cholesterol.

Colon (5 to 24 hours)

Gut flora digest dietary fibre releasing volatile fatty acids, gases and amino acids; also synthesize biotin. Absorption of water, electrolytes and vitamin K.

Mouth

Liver

Gall bladder

Pancreas

Anus

Fig.2.2 The digestive system. The process of digestion and absorption of the major nutrient components of food in different parts of the gut.

of nutrients, such as glucose, fatty acids and amino acids, in the blood should remain relatively constant: a low concentration will be topped up by the release of nutrients from storage sites in the body (the catabolic process of degradation), and a high concentration will be counteracted by the removal of nutrients from the blood into storage forms (the anabolic process of storage). The amount of nutrients in the blood will therefore be dependent on the net balance between the rates of these two processes. In this way, nutrients are always present in the blood and the amount can be increased, very rapidly if required, by altering the rate of each process either separately or both together in opposing directions.

After a meal, the concentrations of glucose, fatty acids and amino acids in the blood will increase considerably as they are absorbed from the gut. The nutrients must then move from the blood into the cells of the body for synthesis into the appropriate storage form.

Similarly, when insufficient nutrients are entering the system, for example, during prolonged food restriction, or when energy demands are increased (such as when you start to run or swim), the body must recognize that energy is required so that the energy stores within the body can be mobilized to maintain the essential energy supply. Otherwise, the concentration of nutrients in the blood will fall dramatically as nutrients are taken up from the blood faster than they are being released from the storage tissues. The potential consequences of confusing the conditions of fed, fasting or exercise would be disastrous.

This fine balance between storing nutrients and breaking them down and mobilizing them to provide energy is called 'turnover' and is controlled by a variety of complex physiological processes involving the liver, the brain and many hormones. It allows the body to make subtle alterations in energy supply to meet the varying demands of extreme endurance, strength or power made upon the body in sport.

Let us consider what happens to carbohydrates, proteins and fats after a meal.

Carbohydrates

The absorption of carbohydrates mainly takes place in the middle section of the small intestine (the jejunum) and the monosaccharides are taken up into the blood. Depending on the metabolic circumstances at the time, there are four possible fates for carbohydrates:

- They may be burned as fuel in the liver to provide the energy needed for the cells of the liver to function normally or used in the synthesis of other compounds.
- If the immediate demand for energy is satisfied, carbohydrates may be stored in the liver as glycogen, to be used for energy at a subsequent point.
- Carbohydrates may be transported as glucose in the blood to other tissues in the body, such as skeletal muscle. These tissues can then either use the glucose as an immediate source of energy or convert it to glycogen.
- If the immediate needs for energy are met and glycogen stores adequately refilled, any excess carbohydrates can be converted to fat to serve as an energy store. However, once carbohydrates have been converted to triglyceride, this cannot be reconverted to glucose in any appreciable amounts.

The amount of energy that can be stored as carbohydrate within the body is relatively limited. Only some 50 kcal/210 kJ are available immediately as glucose within the blood. The liver stores of glycogen will provide approximately 250–300 kcal/1050–1250 kJ, while the glycogen in muscle in the typical adult male will provide about 400–500 kcal/1700–2100 kJ. When these values are compared against the typical expenditure of energy each day of 1500–4000 kcal/6.3–16.8 MJ it is clear that carbohydrates are not a major energy store within the body. They are however, extremely important during exercise. There are several important points to remember about how carbohydrates are used as a fuel:

- The liver must provide glucose for the brain. The central nervous system has an absolute need for glucose as an energy source because it cannot store glycogen itself. If the liver fails to provide sufficient glucose, the supply of energy to the brain will be compromised.
- The concentration of glucose in the blood must be maintained within normal ranges at all times, despite vast differences in the rate at which glucose may enter the blood following a meal or when glucose is being taken up by the muscle during exercise.
- Whereas liver glycogen can be broken down and released into the blood to provide glucose for other tissues, the glycogen within one muscle cannot be mobilized to provide glucose for other tissues (such as the brain or other skeletal muscles).
- The stores of glycogen can **only** be maintained through the continual intake of carbohydrates. They cannot be maintained without adequate carbohydrate supplies — they cannot be synthesized in any appreciable amounts from proteins or from fat.

Proteins

For a long time it was thought that proteins were digested completely — down to free amino acids — before absorption into the blood. Now it is clear, however, that a substantial amount of small peptides, in addition to amino acids, are absorbed by specific transport systems in the latter part of the small intestine called the ileum. The peptides are rapidly hydrolysed (broken down) by enzymes present in the absorptive cells so that only amino acids are found in the portal blood.

The amino acids reaching the liver are not only those consumed in the meal; the amino acids present in the enzymes that digest food and the cells sloughed off from the gut lining are also digested and absorbed. In addition, the mucosal cells of the gut will also interconvert some of the incoming amino acids to others in response to the body's needs. This is important: the

31

body does not wish to waste essential amino acids and recovers them for further use.

There is no storage form of protein as such but the body is continually synthesizing protein from the pool of amino acids within cells and then breaking it down again. While this constant turnover of protein uses considerable amounts of energy, it should not be interpreted as a purely wasteful and futile exercise. The relative balance between the rates of protein synthesis and degradation determines whether protein is deposited within the body or broken down. As it is possible to alter the rates at which protein is independently both synthesized and broken down, extremely fine and subtle alterations in protein metabolism may be achieved.

For example, a net deposition of protein (such as occurs in growth) can be achieved by either increasing the rate of protein synthesis, decreasing the rate of protein degradation or both. Similarly, when amino acids are required to be used for energy (such as in starvation), an increased rate of protein degradation can be achieved by slowing synthesis, increasing breakdown, or both.

There are then three principal fates for protein when amino acids reach the liver:

- Amino acids may be synthesized into proteins, either for structural purposes or as important enzymes, hormones and plasma proteins within the liver.
- They may be released to the blood for subsequent use by other tissues of the body.
- Any amino acids in excess of requirements may be used as an energy source. The process by which glucose is synthesized from amino acids in the liver is called gluconeogenesis. Glucose can also be synthesized from lactate and glycerol by the same process.

The nitrogen part of the amino acid must be removed (a process called deamination) and the resulting carbon skeleton converted to glucose. This may be used either as an immediate energy source or stored as glycogen or triglyceride by either the liver or other tissues such as muscle. The nitrogen waste produced following deamination must not be allowed to accumulate in the body as it is toxic, so it is converted to urea and excreted from the body by the kidneys. As this process also necessitates the excretion of water, the consumption of excessive amounts of protein may compromise fluid balance.

If the total protein stored within the body could be used as energy, some 28,000 kcal/118 MJ would be available, but this is clearly not possible as proteins play many key roles in the body other than as an energy store. Any appreciable losses of protein to provide an energy source will result in a breakdown of skeletal, heart and smooth muscle, reductions in plasma proteins and impairment in immune function, all of which severely affect the well-being of the individual and so must be avoided wherever possible. These functions should only be jeopardized by protein losses as a last resort (for example, when other energy stores are not able to provide sufficient energy such as in starvation).

Fats

Triglycerides are either completely digested to glycerol and three fatty acids or partially digested to a glycerol base with one or two fatty acids still attached. Like amino acids, these are mainly absorbed in the ileum. The way in which fats are absorbed is dependent on the relative size of the fatty acid:

- The smaller, short-chain fatty acids (those less than 10 carbon atoms long) are absorbed directly and are transported to the liver in the blood. On reaching the liver, these fatty acids can either be burnt as fuel or reformed into triglyceride which may be stored in the liver or transported to other cells of the body, packaged in a protein coat as lipoproteins.
- Alternatively, the larger fatty acids are converted back to triglyceride on crossing the cell wall of the gut and enter the lymphatic system as droplets of fat called chylomicrons. In this way, they can enter the general circulation without having to pass through the liver.

Fats may therefore enter the circulation as either lipoproteins or chylomicrons but, before the fatty acids can be taken up by the cells of the body, they must be broken down again to glycerol and fatty acids. The fatty acids can then enter the cells where they may combine with the products of glucose metabolism to reform triglyceride.

In the same way that protein is continually turned over, triglycerides are constantly being synthesized and then broken down. When energy is required, fatty acids may be mobilized from adipose (fatty) tissue and released into the circulation to be delivered to tissues requiring energy by increasing breakdown and decreasing synthesis. The reverse occurs when there is a surfeit of energy in excess of immediate demands: fatty acids and glucose are stored as triglyceride by increasing synthesis and decreasing breakdown.

Unlike carbohydrates and proteins, fats are an ideal energy store. As they are relatively energy-dense, twice as much energy can be stored in 1 g of fat as in 1 g of carbohydrate or protein, and large amounts of energy can be stored in a relatively compact form. In a typical male adult, the fat stores of

33

the body may be equivalent to some 140,000 kcal/590 MJ. People who are relatively fat obviously possess an even greater energy store!

How do we get energy from the body's energy stores?

The mechanisms which convert chemical energy to work must be contained within the millions of cells in the body. Muscle cells, like most cells, require the presence of a substance that can harness energy from the energy-yielding oxidation of foodstuffs and yet can release that energy to the chemical reactions or processes that require it. The most important substance of this type in the human body is adenosine triphosphate (ATP).

ATP — the energy currency

It is important to remember that ATP is not synthesized in one particular tissue and then transported around the body. Instead, every living cell has the capacity to synthesize and use ATP within itself. Also, we do not store energy as ATP — this would be very inefficient and would certainly cause many problems in the control of metabolism as it has been estimated that something like 60–70 kilograms of ATP would be required to complete a marathon!

The molecule of ATP simply consists of a base called adenosine with three phosphate groups joined together in a row — hence the name triphosphate. The energy that is available to be transformed is 'trapped' in the chemical bonds between the three phosphate groups, rather like a chemical spring. In order to liberate the potential energy within the ATP's high-energy phosphate bonds, one of the phosphate groups must be split off leaving just two phosphates, in which form it is called adenosine diphosphate (ADP). So ATP is broken down to ADP whenever energy is required by a specific biological process or reaction.

The amount of ATP within a particular cell is very limited however — probably only enough to cover the energy requirements for a few seconds before becoming depleted. In order to continue to supply ATP, ADP can be reconverted back to ATP again by the addition of another phosphate group. This process of ATP resynthesis requires energy which is generated by the oxidation of carbohydrate, fat and protein within the cell. So ATP can be thought of as the intermediate or common energy currency between the energy store and the reactions or processes requiring energy.

It is very important to appreciate that the processes by which energy is utilized must be tightly coupled with those that produce energy. The harder

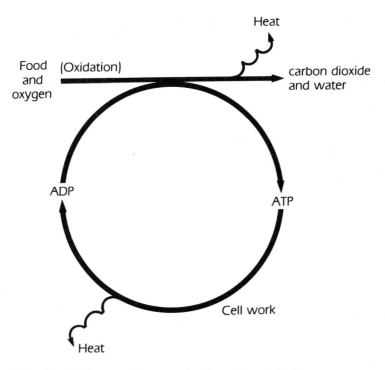

Fig.2.3 Metabolism and heat production. All metabolic processes require energy from the combustion of food and oxygen and they all eventually result in the production of heat (plus carbon dioxide and water). Metabolic rate can be determined by measuring either heat production or oxygen utilization.

you work, the greater the rate at which you use energy and so the faster the rate at which energy must be produced, as is shown in Figure 2.4. Any mismatch between the rates at which ATP is used and the rates at which it is produced will lead to an 'energy crisis' (see page 65) where levels of ATP would fall perilously low. This must be avoided at all costs as without a continual supply of ATP the cell cannot function.

Resynthesizing ATP

So how does the body resynthesize ATP? Muscle cells are well equipped to produce energy, but the amount of energy stored within cells is not sufficient to cover the daily energy needs. Yet the energy stores do allow the cells to produce energy very rapidly when needed and keep pace with requirements until the major energy reserves of the body — the triglycerides

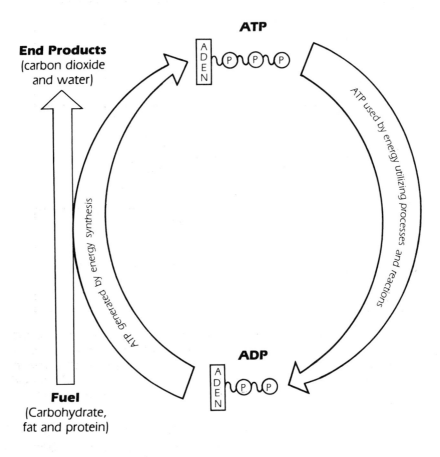

Fig.2.4 The energy cycle. The rate of ATP resynthesis must be tightly coupled with the rate of ATP utilization to avoid a mismatch between the two processes.

stored in the subcutaneous fat cells (under the skin) — can be mobilized and delivered to the working muscle. It would be disastrous if the cells did not possess their own store of energy.

The muscle cells also possess a temporary supply of energy which can be used to resynthesize ATP so that any acute mismatch of production and usage can be alleviated. This is another substance possessing a high-energy phosphate bond called creatine phosphate (CP). When CP is broken down, the energy contained within its high-energy bond can be transferred to ADP to produce ATP. In this way ATP can be resynthesized extremely rapidly — but not indefinitely. The supply of CP is also limited and would only last for 30–60 seconds before becoming depleted if it were the only way of

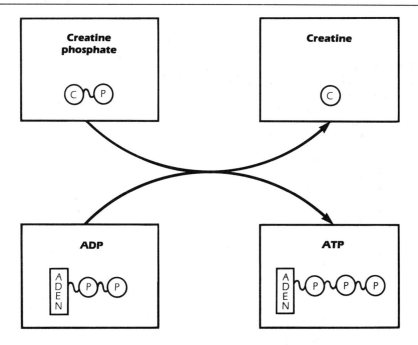

Fig.2.5 ATP resynthesis by creatine phosphate degradation. During exercise when the demand for energy is high, ATP can be regenerated by converting creatine phosphate to creatine. After exercise, the reverse reaction occurs to regenerate creatine phosphate by converting ATP to ADP using ATP released from oxidative metabolism within the mitochondria.

providing more ATP during heavy exercise. Once depleted, the store of CP can only be replenished by reforming the high-energy phosphate bond. The energy required to do this comes from the oxidation of foodstuffs, which can only occur when the rate at which energy is produced exceeds the rate at which it is used — part of the recovery process after the exercise task has been completed.

Mitochondria: 'powerhouses' in the cells

Despite the variety of energy sources (fuel) in the diet, the energy used during exercise is primarily derived from the carbohydrate and fat stores of the body. Protein may also be used to some extent, especially under conditions where the supply of carbohydrate is particularly limited or during prolonged endurance exercise. Carbohydrates, fats and proteins are initially broken down to produce energy within muscle cells in different ways which depends on the rate at which energy is required and the amount of fuel that

Mitochondrion (in section)   Mitochondria (in section)

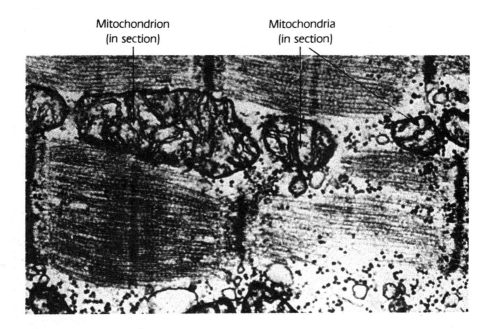

Fig.2.6 Electronmicrograph of mitochondria within a muscle cell.

is available (see later). However, the ultimate fate of all fuel is to be combusted in the presence of oxygen to release energy which can then be trapped by ATP as well as carbon dioxide and water.

The process of oxidation occurs within highly specialized structures within the cells called mitochondria. These structures have been called the 'engines' or 'powerhouses' of the cells and account for most of the oxygen consumed by the body. The main function of the mitochondria within the cell is to take up specific intermediates of carbohydrate, fat and protein metabolism, along with oxygen and ADP, and generate energy in the form of ATP by a specific metabolic pathway called the Krebs cycle (named after Sir Hans Krebs who did so much to identify it). So the Krebs cycle is a major focal point of metabolism — the common pathway for the conversion of the various forms of chemical energy in the diet (nutrients) to the common currency of energy in the body (ATP).

Energy from carbohydrates

The principal role of carbohydrates within the body is as a source of energy. They have certain advantages: they are capable of rapid release from storage and are the only fuel that can be used to generate very high rates of energy production when the oxidative processes are insufficient. In addition to the

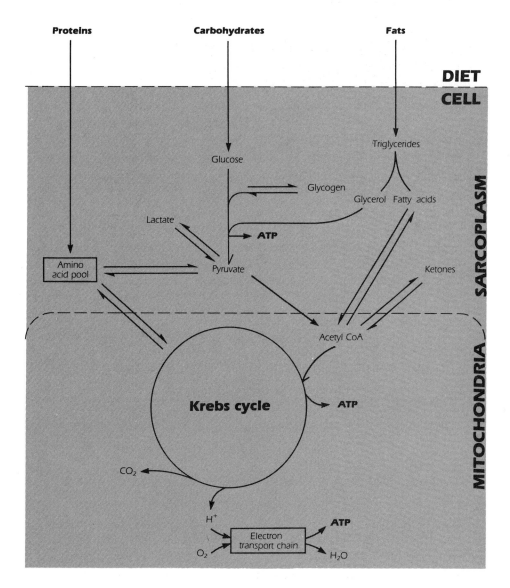

Fig.2.7 The multiple fates of nutrients in the body.

store of glycogen within the muscle, the glycogen stored within the liver may also be used to provide glucose. This can then be taken up by the muscle to supplement its own supplies of carbohydrate, particularly as the stores of glycogen within the muscle become depleted.

Anaerobic metabolism

At the beginning of exercise or when energy demand rate is high (such as during a sprint), the rate at which energy is required exceeds the rate at which the oxidative processes can generate ATP by fully combusting carbohydrate. Glycogen is initially broken down to a smaller compound called pyruvate which can then be oxidized by the Krebs cycle. However, under conditions where energy is required rapidly, the glycogen within the muscle can be incompletely broken down by converting the pyruvate to a substance called lactic acid. This process takes place outside the mitochondria and does not require oxygen — hence it is often referred to as **anaerobic** metabolism (that is, without oxygen). Although the amount of ATP generated for each unit of glycogen used is very small (only 2 units of ATP per unit of glycogen used), this inefficient process does allow energy to be produced extremely rapidly and so keep pace with the rate at which energy is needed.

So, under conditions where the rate of ATP generation is important, rather than the total production of energy over a prolonged period — such as during power sports and most field games (soccer, hockey, rugby, etc) — the ability to generate ATP by lactic acid formation is extremely important. But, once again this process cannot continue indefinitely. Within the muscle cell, the lactic acid breaks down to produce lactate and hydrogen ions. Unless these hydrogen ions are removed from the cell, they will accumulate, making the contents of the muscle cell extremely acidic. If allowed to proceed unabated, this would lead eventually to the destruction of the cell, so the production of lactate and hydrogen ions, and therefore ATP by this process must be restricted to tolerable levels (see page 68).

In contrast to the relatively small amounts of ATP generated per unit of glycogen used outside the mitochondria, considerably greater amounts of ATP can be generated when carbohydrate is oxidized completely within the mitochondria ie, during **aerobic** metabolism (with oxygen). As this process requires oxygen, the supply and uptake of oxygen to the working muscle must be suitably accelerated by increasing ventilation and cardiac output resulting in an increased delivery of oxygen to the mitochondria. For each glucose unit, either from the glycogen within the muscle or delivered to the muscle from the liver, that is completely oxidized, 36–38 units of ATP are generated in comparison to the 2 units of ATP generated under conditions of lactic acid formation. Therefore, producing energy by lactate formation may be extremely rapid, but it is highly uneconomical in that it will use up the glycogen stores very quickly. Consequently, anything that alters the relative amount of glycogen that is either oxidized or converted to lactic acid would have a considerable impact upon the total amount of energy derived from the store of glycogen. This is particularly important where the continued supply of glycogen may be the most important factor limiting performance.

Lactate formation: new ideas

It was originally believed that lactate formation only occurred under conditions where the supply of oxygen was unavailable. This concept of purely anaerobic energy production was derived from early studies examining the energy production in muscles of frogs where the supply of oxygen to the working muscle was stopped or from the fermentation of yeasts in sealed containers. Under such circumstances, the energy to support the frog muscle cell or yeast could be produced by forming lactate. But, while a lack of oxygen will result in lactate formation, not all lactate is formed only because of an insufficient oxygen supply. It is now becoming more widely accepted that the rate at which lactate is produced is directly related to the rate at which energy is being produced.

One other important point that should not be overlooked is that lactate is not a metabolic dead-end and its formation does not mean that all the potential energy stored within the carbohydrate has been wasted. There are several possible fates for lactate, once formed, which would result in a removal or clearance of lactate from the system:

- It may be converted back to pyruvate within the same muscle cell when the rate of energy provision from oxidative metabolism is sufficient to meet the demands for energy. This would then spare glucose units from glycogen within the muscle as well as entry of glucose from the circulation, as the pyruvate that is formed could then be oxidized in place of pyruvate formed from glucose or glycogen.
- Lactate may leave the muscle cell to be taken up by other muscle cells within the same muscle. Such cells may have exhausted their own supply of glycogen and be in need of suitable carbohydrate to convert back to pyruvate and then either oxidize to produce energy, or use to rebuild the glycogen store of the cell.
- Alternatively, lactate may leave the muscle and be taken up by the liver and converted back to glucose. The glucose formed by this process can then be released back into the blood to be taken up by the muscle cell as further fuel for either energy production or glycogen repletion.

Therefore while the eventual metabolic fate of any lactate formed will be oxidation, the immediate fate will depend on the energetic demands on the cell prevailing at that time.

The idea that the cell suddenly switches over from aerobic to anaerobic metabolism is therefore no longer tenable. Lactate formation during exercise now appears to be directly proportional to the rate at which energy is being produced and does not start suddenly at a certain point or threshold of exercise intensity (an 'anaerobic threshold'). Instead lactate is being produced continually and only accumulates when the rate at which it is produced exceeds the rate at which it can be cleared from the system.

Energy from fats

The stages by which triglycerides stored within the adipose tissue of the body or the muscle cells are converted into energy within the muscle cells are multiple:

- The first is to mobilize the triglyceride store within the adipose tissue and bring about the release of free fatty acids into the circulation. This process is under the control of several hormones, the most important of which are adrenaline and noradrenaline which are released when energy is required. These hormones are often known as the 'fight or flight' hormones in that they prepare the body for exercise.
- Once the free fatty acids are released into the circulation they are transported, in association with a carrier protein called albumin, to the working muscle. The glycerol that is also released is taken up by the liver in order to be converted to glucose by a process called gluconeogenesis (see page 60).
- The release of fatty acids from the adipose tissue and the increased blood flow results in fatty acids entering the muscle. (The uptake of fatty acids by skeletal muscle is directly related to the concentration of free fatty acids in the blood and the rate of blood flowing through the capillaries of the muscle.) These fatty acids may either join the fatty acids released from the intramuscular stores of triglyceride, be oxidized immediately or be stored as triglyceride within the muscle.
- The first stage of the oxidation of fatty acids requires both energy and the activation of the fatty acid, so this step uses ATP. These activated fatty acids are then transported into the mitochondria via a special carrier mechanism. Along with the delivery of fatty acids to the muscle (above), this is believed to be one of the most crucial stages in determining the rate at which fatty acids may be used as an energy source. Clearly, the greater the number of mitochondria present within the cell, the greater the capacity to take up fatty acids and oxidize them to produce energy.

● Once in the mitochondria, the activated fatty acids are broken down further so that they may then enter the Krebs cycle and be oxidized in the same way as carbohydrate. The number of ATP units generated by the process depends on the number of carbon atoms present in the fatty acid chain — the longer the fatty acid, the greater the number of ATP units that will be generated. As the majority of fatty acids range in length from 10 to 24 carbon atoms, the energy yield per unit of fatty acid is considerable (about 80–200 ATP units).

So, whereas only 36–38 ATP units are generated by glucose oxidation, the potential energy yield during fatty acid oxidation is much greater. Consequently, any factor which increases the rate of fatty acid oxidation would have a considerable impact upon the total amount of energy generated. However, the primary limitation to the rate of energy resynthesis from fat is that it is dependent upon oxidation within the mitochondria: while the yield is great in absolute amounts, the **rate** at which ATP is resynthesized is comparatively low.

Some tissues (such as the heart and liver) are well suited for energy resynthesis from fat oxidation but others (such as the brain and red blood cells) are dependent on glycolysis to provide energy and are totally dependent on the supply and utilization of glucose. Skeletal muscle, on the other hand, is ideally equipped to handle a whole variety of different fuels, although the capacity to oxidize fatty acids does vary considerably between the different types of muscle fibre. Those fibres with a high oxidative capacity (large numbers of mitochondria) and good blood supply — the Type I or SO fibres — are better able to oxidize fatty acids than the Type IIb or FG fibres, which are better suited to generating energy from carbohydrate metabolism (see page 47).

Ketones

There is another form of fat that can be used to provide energy. Under extreme conditions (for example, prolonged exercise, starvation or in diabetes), the excess free fatty acids released into the circulation are converted by the liver to ketones. Apart from being a suitable fuel for energy metabolism in the muscle, ketones are particularly important as they are the only other source of energy (apart from glucose) that can be used by the brain and nervous tissue. Ketones are taken up by the brain and skeletal muscle and enter the Krebs cycle to be oxidized to produce ATP.

Energy from proteins

It was originally believed that proteins, because of their important role in the structure and function of the body, were spared as an energy source wherever possible. More recently, though, studies have demonstrated that during prolonged exercise, amino acids are metabolized as an energy source along with carbohydrates and fats. Apart from simply providing energy, amino acids are of particular importance in that they may be metabolized to glucose (through gluconeogenesis) and can therefore provide glucose for those tissues which have to rely on it as an energy source and support the oxidation of other fuels such as fats.

Before it can be used as energy, the nitrogen part of the amino acid must be removed (by a process called deamination) and converted to ammonia, leaving the remainder of the amino acid — the carbon skeleton — to be used as an energy source. The majority of carbon skeletons resulting from deamination form either pyruvate or one of the Krebs cycle intermediates. In this form they can easily enter into the oxidative pathway and be used to generate ATP within the mitochondria. (The ammonia generated by this process must be removed from the body as, accumulated, it is extremely hazardous. Converted to urea within the liver, the ammonia can be released into the blood and transported to the kidney from where it can be excreted in the urine.)

There are three principal fates for the carbon skeleton after deamination:

- The carbon atoms may be converted to glucose to be used to support those tissues which are dependent on it. This gluconeogenic process (the making of new glucose, see page 60) is especially important as it allows the liver to maintain its supply of glucose to tissues such as the brain, even when its own stores of glycogen may be low. For example, the liver cannot store sufficient glycogen to cover totally the demands for glucose overnight — irrespective of how much food was consumed the previous day. So, in order to ensure that the supply of glucose to the circulation matches its removal, increasing the rate of glucose production from gluconeogenesis provides sufficient glucose until more nutrients become available at breakfast. In the same way, the glycerol released into the circulation with free fatty acids can be taken up by the liver and converted to glucose by this process.
- The carbon skeletons may be used as an energy source for those tissues where the internal store of carbohydrate is reduced. In addition to simply providing energy, they also make it possible to supply the additional Krebs cycle intermediates required to replace those that have been lost from the cycle. These would normally be maintained from carbohydrate metabolism but, as glycogen stores become depleted and

that rate of carbohydrate metabolism is reduced, an alternative supply of Krebs cycle intermediates is advantageous. Unless the supply of these intermediates is maintained, it is not possible for the Krebs cycle to continue generating ATP from other substrates, such as fatty acids, if carbohydrate stores are limited.

● Under conditions where the supply of glucose exceeds the requirement for energy, the carbon skeletons may be converted to fatty acids and stored as triglyceride.

Summary

■ Energy is stored within the body mainly as glycogen (carbo-hydrate) and triglyceride (fat), and energy is derived from carbo-hydrate, fat, protein and alcohol within the food that we eat.

■ Adenosine triphosphate (ATP) serves to transfer the energy derived from the oxidation of foodstuffs within the mitochondria of cells to the chemical reactions and processes that require energy by the formation and breaking of a phosphate bond.

■ The amount of ATP available within the cell is limited. In order to prevent the depletion of ATP, the processes by which ATP is generated must be tightly coupled with the processes that use ATP.

■ Creatine phosphate can be used to regenerate ATP to alleviate any acute mismatching in the production and usage of ATP, yet supply is limited.

■ The harder you work, the greater the rate of ATP utilization, and the greater the rate of ATP resynthesis.

■ Energy can be derived from the oxidation of intramuscular stores (glycogen and triglyceride) or substrates delivered to the working muscle by the blood (eg, glucose, free fatty acids, ketones or branchchain amino acids). Energy can also be derived from the incomplete combustion of intramuscular glycogen to lactic acid — anaerobic glycolysis.

- Whereas the total energy yield from anaerobic glycolysis is small compared to that gained by oxidation of either fat or carbohydrate, the **rate** at which ATP can be resynthesized is very great but must be restricted to tolerable levels.

- The formation of lactic acid is not a metabolic dead-end — lactate may be reconverted back to pyruvate and oxidized in place of pyruvate derived from glucose or glycogen during exercise — thus sparing glycogen.

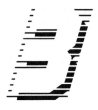 # Energy into muscular activity

How is energy used during exercise?

In order to carry out any form of muscular work, the muscles of the body must contract so as to generate force. In most situations the length of the muscle will shorten considerably and, when these forces are applied through joints, a limb will move. This type of muscular work is called an isotonic or isokinetic contraction. In other situations, no discernible shortening of muscle will be visible yet a force will be generated — an isometric contraction. In both instances, though, the cells of the muscle generate force by shortening in length: this process requires energy.

Muscle fibres

Skeletal muscle tissue is composed primarily of different combinations of individual muscle cells (fibres) and of connective tissue. Connective tissue runs from one end of the muscle to the other, existing within the muscle tissue surrounding the fibres and giving rise to bundles of fibres called fasciculi (see Figure 3.1). In some muscles, these fibres run longitudinally (along the length of the muscle), while in others, such as the gastrocnemius (a calf muscle), they are attached to connective tissue within the muscle and consequently do not run exactly in the direction of the muscle tissue.

The various types of skeletal muscle fibres can be classified either on the basis of their speed of contraction (known as their twitch characteristics), their resistance to fatigue or their metabolic characteristics. Muscle fibres within human skeletal muscle are usually identified by using histochemical techniques (that is, testing chemical reactions on tissues) on samples of muscle. The fibres are placed in various solutions which induce chemical reactions resulting in different stains depending on the metabolic characteristics of the fibre.

Three main types of skeletal muscle fibre have been identified in man on the basis of twitch and metabolic characteristics:

● The Type I (slow twitch) fibre, which is red in colour, slow to contract, relatively resistant to fatigue and has a high oxidative capacity (that is, a

47

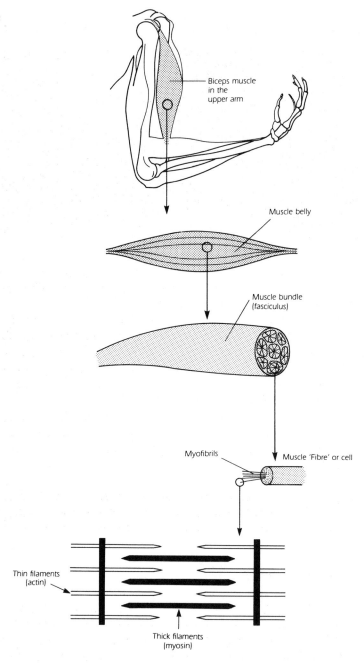

Biceps muscle
in the
upper arm

Muscle belly

Muscle bundle
(fasciculus)

Myofibrils

Muscle 'Fibre' or cell

Thin filaments
(actin)

Thick filaments
(myosin)

Fig.3.1 The structure of human skeletal muscle under increasing strengths of magnification.

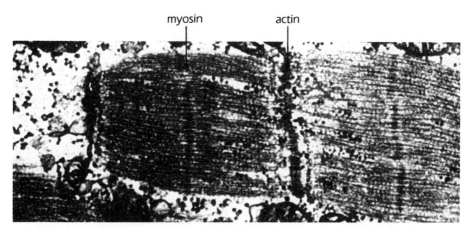

myosin   actin

Fig.3.2 Electron micrograph of actin and myosin protein

high potential to generate ATP by the oxidation of carbohydrate, fat and protein within the mitochondria). Because of these characteristics it is generally termed the slow oxidative (SO) fibre.

- The Type II (fast twitch) fibre, divided into Type IIa and Type IIb according to oxidative capacity and resistance to fatigue. The Type IIb fibre is the classical fast twitch fibre, appearing white in colour; it is fast to contract yet fatigues rapidly. It possesses a relatively low oxidative capacity, yet a very high capacity to generate ATP by glycolysis. It is generally termed the fast glycolytic (FG) fibre.
- The Type IIa fibre is an intermediate between the SO and FG fibres, being fast to contract, relatively fatigue-resistant and possessing a high oxidative and glycolytic capacity. It is generally termed the fast oxidative glycolytic (FOG) fibre.

Although physical training can significantly affect the metabolic characteristics of skeletal muscle (and consequently the histochemical appearance of muscle cells), muscle fibre type is primarily determined by hereditary factors.

Muscle fibre recruitment

The recruitment (bringing into action) of these fibres during muscular work generally follows a hierarchical pattern: starting with the SO fibres, then the FOG fibres and, last and less frequently, the FG fibres. Recruitment is generally determined not just by the speed of movement but also the force necessary to perform the movement. For example, for rapid lifting of a very light weight, the SO fibres may be recruited exclusively, whereas all the muscle

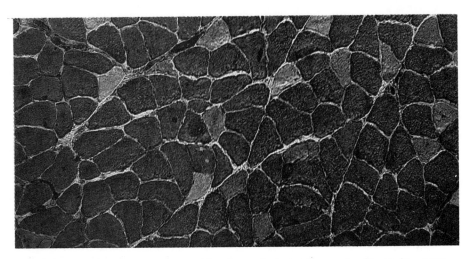

Fig.3.3 A low power magnification of skeletal muscle fibres in cross section.

fibres will be recruited for lifting a very heavy weight, which must of necessity be moved slowly.

It is also important to note that, as most muscles of the body are a mixture of these different muscle fibres, not all of the muscle will be recruited during muscular work. Selective recruitment of one type of fibre population may occur and the remaining fibres be recruited less often. Also, not all of one fibre population is recruited simultaneously; at any one time, some fibres will be actively participating in the generation of force, others will have been working but are now fatigued, while some have yet to be recruited. Consequently, a selective dropping out of fibres may occur during the course of an exercise task as fibres become fatigued, resulting in a reduction in the total number of fibres that can be recruited to perform that particular task.

How the muscle fibre contracts: actin and myosin

If you view skeletal muscle under high magnification, the fibres appear to be striped. This is because of the presence of the myofibrils — the two main proteins of contraction (or contractile proteins) called actin and myosin (see Figure 3.2). It is the interaction of these two contractile proteins (resulting from a series of complex events which require energy) that leads to the contraction of the muscle fibre and muscular movement.

When a nerve impulse is relayed to the muscle, a change in the electrical properties of the cell surface spreads this signal to the whole fibre. Calcium ions are released into the sarcoplasm (the fluid space within the cell), which provides the stimulus for the actin and myosin to interact.

The sliding filament theory

The exact process by which energy produces an interaction of actin and myosin which shortens the muscle fibre is not fully understood, though one explanation is provided by the so-called 'sliding filament' theory. This suggests that:

- In the resting state, the ATP combines with myosin to energize it so that the head of the myosin filament is like a loaded and cocked revolver ready to discharge.
- When calcium ions are released into the sarcoplasm, changes in the actin filament produce a site where the two filaments may bind together to form a cross-bridge.

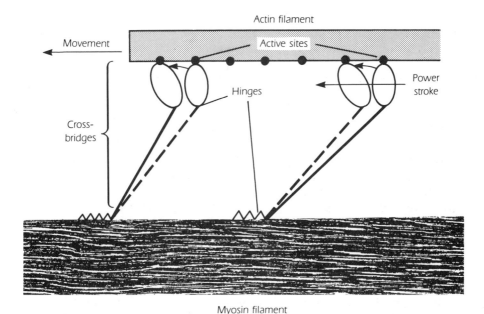

Fig.3.4 Sliding Filament Theory
Muscle contraction (shortening) is thought to occur when cross-bridges extend from myosin to actin and a conformational change occurs in the cross-bridge. The specifics of this schematic model are yet to be worked out. (SOURCE: Modified from H.E. Huxley. 1958.)

51

- The binding of actin to myosin triggers the release of potential energy stored within the myosin head, resulting in movement; the release of heat as energy is transformed from chemical energy to mechanical work.
- This involves the splitting of one of the phosphate groups from the ATP to form ADP, which lowers the supply of ATP for subsequent work.
- The protruding heads of the myosin filaments interact with the actin filaments and the contraction occurs as the result of a ratchet or oarlike movement between the two filaments — the myosin filaments actually appear to walk up the actin.

In order for the muscle to contract further or relax, the cross-bridge must be broken and the myosin re-energized. This requires the presence of ATP, again firstly to bind to myosin to energize and secondly to pump the calcium ions from the sarcoplasm back into the storage sites ready for the next contraction.

Energy is also required to re-establish the resting concentrations of sodium and potassium on either side of the muscle cell membranes (these were altered as the electrical signal spread throughout the muscle during contraction). Similarly, any reduction in the amount of high-energy phosphates within the cells must also be replaced.

The muscle and energy

In the context of exercise, thousands of muscle cells will contract at the same split second — and every time a muscle contracts energy is used and ATP is changed to ADP. The stores of ATP within the muscle are extremely small so further supplies must be resynthesized immediately. Also, the rate at which ATP is resynthesized must keep pace with the rate at which it is being used: any mismatch between the rates of resynthesis and utilization will result in either a reduction or an increase in the amount of ATP within the muscle cell, either of which would be highly damaging to its integrity and function.

Many of the energy reactions within the cell are controlled by the relative concentrations of ATP and ADP within it. Changes in the amount of ATP or ADP (or both in opposite directions) provide a sensitive means of determining whether more or less ATP should be resynthesized and couples the supply of substrates with the energy needs of the cell. A reduction in the availability of ATP within the cell would impair the function of many of the essential physiological and metabolic processes necessary to support life, so the concentrations of ATP and ADP must be maintained at a constant level wherever possible.

The key to how the muscle copes with the vastly differing demands it faces, both in everyday life and in sport, lies in:

● How the various substrates available to the muscle are integrated;
● The proportions in which they are used (relative utilization).

At rest

Even at rest the muscle is not totally inactive. Small adjustments in posture and tone require muscle recruitment and energy utilization; the turnover of protein, carbohydrate and fat within the cell and the pumping of ions all require energy. As the rate of ATP utilization is relatively slow at rest, sufficient ATP can be resynthesized by oxidative combustion of fat. This requires little carbohydrate which is derived primarily from the glycogen stores within the muscle, so relatively little glucose is taken up by the muscle from the circulation.

Exercise begins

In contrast, as soon as the muscle starts to perform muscular work, the rate at which ATP is utilized (and hence required) is increased enormously. During maximal exercise, such as during a sprint, ATP utilization may, within seconds, have to rise one-thousand-fold over that observed at rest. This demands a rapid and immediate increase in the rate at which ATP is resynthesized in order to prevent a rapid drop in ATP concentrations within the cell; as the acceleration of oxidative metabolism is relatively slow, some other form of ATP resynthesis is required. The stores of CP within the muscle serve to provide the necessary rate of ATP resynthesis but these stores are also fairly small, probably sufficient to support 10–15 seconds of maximal exercise. They merely serve as an energy buffer intended to make good any temporary deficits in ATP resynthesis; they are not a longterm energy store and they fall considerably at the onset of exercise.

Exercise continues

As exercise proceeds, the massive mobilization of glycogen leads to a rapid increase in the supply of pyruvate for oxidation. This 'avalanche' of energy-supplying substrate exceeds the rate of entry of pyruvate into the mitochondria for oxidation and results in an accumulation of glycolytic intermediates (between glycogen and pyruvate) effectively backing up in the pathway. This serves to inhibit the uptake of glucose into the cell, so blood glucose is spared. If glucose uptake was not inhibited, the muscle's capacity to utilize glucose would drain the circulation of glucose within minutes. However, the supply of energy can be maintained by converting pyruvate to lactate, thereby maintaining ATP resynthesis.

As ventilation and cardiac output increase with the challenge of exercise, more oxygen is delivered to the working muscle and the mitochondria can more effectively oxidize the available substrate. This results in a greater entry of pyruvate into the mitochondria from the intermediates within the pathway, from further intermediates formed from glycogen and from the potential pyruvate available as lactate. In this way, a greater proportion of the total ATP resynthesis shifts from CP utilization and lactate formation to the oxidation of pyruvate, reducing the rate at which glycogen is being broken down.

The reduction in glycolytic intermediates (between glycogen and pyruvate) makes it possible to utilize the glucose being released from the liver (as a result of the hormonal stimulation of liver glycogen degradation), so a greater proportion of the energy supply can now come from glucose oxidation. However, the rate at which glucose is taken up by the working muscle must not exceed the rate at which it is being released from the liver or a reduction in blood glucose will occur. Similarly, the delivery of fatty acids from the circulation will also increase as fatty acids are released into the blood and as relatively more of the cardiac output is made available to the muscle. Thus, a greater proportion of the rate of ATP resynthesis will move to fat oxidation as exercise proceeds.

At steady-state

Eventually, after 5–15 minutes, a steady-state situation develops whereby the body has adjusted to the increased demand for ATP by increasing the delivery and utilization of substrate to match the rate at which energy is being used. During prolonged exercise performed at a relatively constant pace and rate of energy demand, the desired rate of ATP resynthesis is maintained by oxidizing a mixture of carbohydrates (both as glycogen within the muscle and as glucose delivered from the liver) and fats (both within the muscle and delivered to the muscle as free fatty acids).

This increased supply of ATP (derived from oxidative metabolism within mitochondria) in excess of requirements may also make it possible to resynthesize the CP pool that may have been depleted at the onset of exercise. In addition, the body's thermoregulatory system will eventually adjust to accommodate the increase in heat production and the body temperature will level off, slightly elevated.

Beyond steady-state

During exercise, once this steady-state has been attained, any further increases in the rate of ATP utilization must be accommodated immediately. If a runner comes to a hill, for example, the increase in energy requirement will depend on the incline of the hill and the speed at which the runner attempts the hill. If the rise in ATP requirement is relatively small, this may be met by simply increasing the rate at which ATP is resynthesized from oxidative metabolism. However, if the gradient is great and the pace maintained, then a fall in ATP concentration within the cell may be alleviated by increasing lactate formation and CP utilization. The lactate accumulation and CP depletion accrued during the climb may be accommodated once the rate of ATP utilization decreases (for example, when running down hill) or if oxidative metabolism can be sufficiently accelerated. However, if the extent of this lactate accumulation and CP depletion is too great or ignored then fatigue may result.

Similarly, when the body must work at greater exercise intensities than can be supported by oxidative metabolism alone, the body does not attain a steady-state. Instead, the accumulation of lactate exceeds the rate at which it can be cleared, glycogen stores are rapidly utilized in preference to fats or glucose and CP stores will also be depleted.

Substrates: integration and control

The success of the muscles' response to a wide range of demands involves these important points:

- A mixture of different substrates or fuels is used at any one time. The muscles do not use one form of substrate exclusively and change to another when the first becomes depleted (for example, switching from carbohydrates to fats once glycogen stores are empty).
- The body draws preferentially upon the greatest store of energy available — fat — to provide the bulk of ATP is resynthesis; this is logical as the amount of energy available from other sources is relatively small. However, despite the vast amount of energy available in fat, the **rate** at which fat oxidation takes place to provide energy is relatively limited. The difference between the rate of ATP production and ATP utilization is made up by using carbohydrate and CP — effectively topping up the rate of ATP synthesis. It is this integration and control of substrate utilization that makes it possible for humans to perform such amazing athletic feats. From studies on ultradistance runners it has been estimated that only exercise intensities up to approximately 50 per cent

55

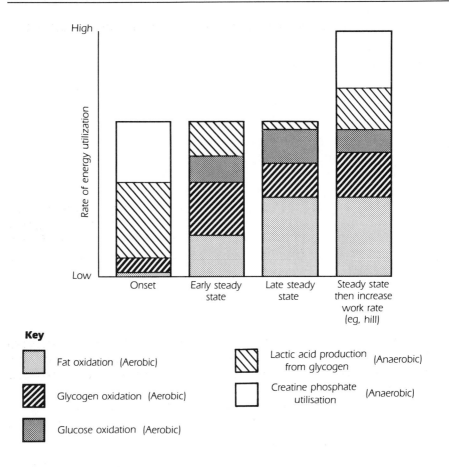

Fig.3.5 Changes in the type of 'fuel' used to provide energy at the onset of exercise and during exercise.

VO$_2$max can be supported by fat oxidation alone. Any activities at greater exercise intensities will require a significant contribution to ATP resynthesis from carbohydrate metabolism. As most sports are performed at exercise intensities of greater than 75 per cent V̇O$_2$max, they are clearly dependent on carbohydrate.

Which fuels are used during exercise?

The integration of all the various substrates must be finely controlled in order to deal with the vast range of demands imposed by different types of sport.

Five principal factors dictate the relative utilization of fuel during exercise:

- Intensity of exercise task
- Duration of exercise task
- Type of exercise
- Training status of the individual
- Preceding diet

Exercise intensity

Low intensity

At low exercise intensities, such as a jog, the rate at which energy must be resynthesized is also relatively low and can be met by simultaneously oxidizing a mixture of fat, glucose and glycogen. Some carbohydrate must be used, though, as the body simply cannot produce energy fast enough by oxidising fat only.

Submaximal intensity

In contrast, when working at exercise intensities just below or comparable to maximal aerobic capacity that is, 90–100 per cent $\dot{V}O_2$max (eg, fast run), the energy demands are so great and energy is required so quickly that the balance is shifted to predominantly carbohydrate. The oxidation of fats and carbohydrate alone cannot meet the rates at which ATP must be resynthesized, so lactate formation, in combination with carbohydrate oxidation, will provide the bulk of the energy resynthesis.

Maximal intensity

When working at truly maximal rates (eg, fast sprint), the contribution of oxidative metabolism is relatively minor and the majority of energy resynthesis is derived from CP utilization and lactate formation. Consequently, the duration of activity is limited as fatigue occurs rapidly. During sprinting, the rate of energy utilization goes up six-hundred to one-thousand-fold and results in rapidly accelerating glycogen mobilization in an attempt to maintain the rates of energy resynthesis. If it were possible to maintain indefinitely the rates of glycogen mobilization observed over the initial seconds of maximal effort, the entire glycogen store could be depleted within 60 seconds. (These same glycogen stores would be sufficient to maintain energy provision over several hours of a marathon.) However, it is not possible to continue working at such rates and the sprinter slows considerably as fatigue occurs.

To conclude, the harder you exercise the greater the rate at which you use up your glycogen stores (See Figure 3.6).

Exercise duration

How long you can exercise will clearly be related to how hard you are exercising, so intensity is probably the most important factor dictating substrate utilization. However, if the exercise intensity is maintained at a constant level, such as during endurance exercise lasting several hours, then the duration of exercise will alter the relative mixture of fuel combusted.

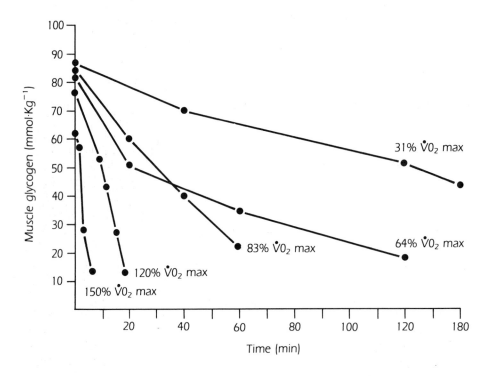

Fig.3.6. Glycogen depletion from the lateral portion of the quadriceps femoris muscle in bicycle exercise of different intensities and durations. The lightest workload results in some depletion of muscle glycogen. However, the most rapid and greatest glycogen depletion occurs with short-term, intense exercise. (Adapted from Gollnick, et al 1974.)

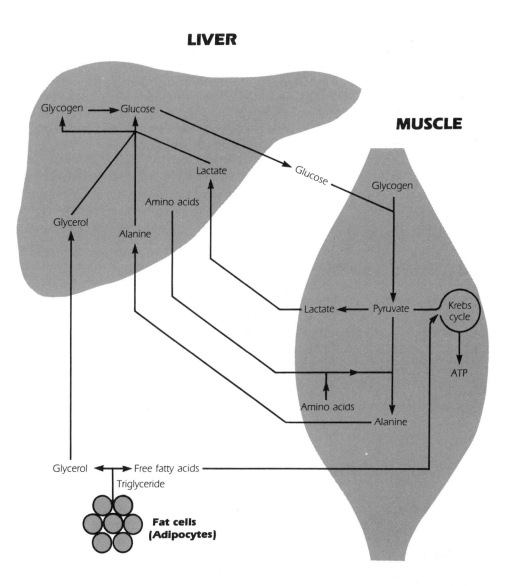

Fig.3.7 Gluconeogenesis. The liver is capable of synthesizing glucose from fat stores to support energy metabolism in the exercising muscles. The process is represented in a simplified form in the diagram above.

Glycogen declines

At the onset of endurance exercise, after steady-state has been attained (that is, when the runner has settled down to a steady pace), glycogen within the muscle will probably provide about 50–60 per cent of the total energy resynthesis, with the remainder primarily from free fatty acids with some glucose uptake. Then, as exercise proceeds and the stores of glycogen decrease, the utilization of glycogen declines and fats become the primary substrate, approximately 60 per cent of the total energy utilization. Meanwhile, there is a shift towards glucose as the source of carbohydrate to maintain the desired rate of ATP resynthesis and utilization.

Gluconeogenesis

So there is a move away from intramuscular stores of energy to the much larger energy stores outside the muscle. Although the size of the liver glycogen store would not provide much energy in the form of glucose in itself, the capacity of the liver to synthesize glucose from other sources during exercise is considerable. This process of gluconeogenesis whereby the end-products of mobilizing fatty acids and glycolysis are taken up by the liver to produce glucose, is of prime importance. The substances contributing to gluconeogenesis, such as glycerol (produced when triglycerides are broken down to release free fatty acids) and lactate, pyruvate and alanine (released from the working muscle as glycolysis proceeds), are converted to glucose and this can then be released back into the blood and taken up by the working muscle to provide energy.

Other substrates

In addition, as the carbohydrate reserves of the muscle become limited, the capacity of the muscle to take up and utilize amino acids as an energy source increases — in particular the branched-chain amino acids: leucine, isoleucine and valine. So too does the capacity to utilize ketone bodies produced by the liver from the excess of fatty acids available in the circulation.

So, as exercise proceeds, there is a progressive shift away from glycogen towards other substrates, but the potential rate at which energy may be resynthesized without using glycogen is limited and decreases considerably as exercise goes on. If the rate at which energy may be resynthesized does not keep pace with the rate at which it is being used, then the exercise intensity must be reduced in order to prevent an energy crisis occurring.

Adjustment in exercise intensity

Failure to recognize the need for adjustment will lead to such acute fatigue that, rather than simply slowing down, the body will be forced to stop exercising completely.

An example of such an adjustment in exercise intensity is the way in which the running speed of competitors settles after the first two days of ultra-distance events (such as the seven-day races). After an initial drop in pace over the first 24–48 hours, they then settle into a pace which they can maintain for the rest of the race. After the first day, the contributions made by glycogen metabolism are likely to be minimal, so this pace (around 50 per cent of the runner's $\dot{V}O_2max$) is probably equivalent to the rate of energy utilization that can be met by fatty acid oxidation and gluconeogenesis alone. This explains why pace judgement is so critical during endurance events.

Exercise type

The type of exercise — whether performed continuously, or as periods of exercise interspersed with periods of recovery or lowered exercise intensity (intermittent exercise) — will also influence the choice and rates of substrate utilization.

Most team games are good examples of intermittent activity. If an activity is performed intermittently much lower rates of glycogen utilization will be observed than if the same amount of exercise is performed continuously without recovery periods. In relatively brief high-intensity periods of exercise, the lower rate of glycogen depletion may be due to a greater oxidative utilization of glycogen (less lactate formation) or a greater CP utilization in each bout, as the recovery period between bouts would allow the oxygen stores of the muscle to be recharged and CP to be resynthesized. In contrast, when lower-intensity of exercise is performed intermittently over prolonged periods, the glycogen-sparing effect may be the result of a greater fat utilization, lactate clearance or glycogen repletion during recovery.

One feature of intermittent exercise is that recovery periods between bouts enable more work to be performed as the consequences of fatigue are then less notable. The concentration of lactate in the blood is much lower when work is performed intermittently so, while there is a tendency to spare glycogen during intermittent exercise, more glycogen may be utilized in total as more work is performed.

Training status

Endurance training also results in lower rates of glycogen utilization for the same work, achieved through a greater oxidative utilization of glycogen (less glycogen being accumulated as lactate) and a greater proportion of the total energy requirement being met by the oxidation of fats and other substrates, such as ketones and amino acids. This situation results from metabolic and physiological changes which serve to increase the oxidative capacity of the working muscle, including:

- A greater density of mitochondria within the cell, leading to an increase in oxidative enzymes
- Increased capillarization — more capillaries supplying blood to each muscle cell
- Enhanced gluconeogenic capacities of both liver and muscle
- A greater proportion of cardiac output that can be distributed to the working muscle.

So, the point at which glycogen becomes limiting and contributes to the fatigue process is delayed.

One very noticeable effect of training is that, by bringing about these changes, it makes the same task easier to perform. However, in most competitive situations there is little desire to finish in a better condition in the same time or for the same degree of effort. Instead, it is more likely that more work is desired — such that the rate of work is increased to a comparable point of fatigue or discomfort.

How training enhances performance

Training appears to expand the individual's capacity for oxidative metabolism and produces a more economical utilization of energy stores. So, following training for any given amount of activity and rate of energy utilization, relatively more of the required rate of energy resynthesis can be met by oxidative processes (and fat oxidation in particular). But the capacity to increase the rate of energy resynthesis further through the same potential for glycogen metabolism, and thus produce an even greater rate of energy utilization is still available. Therefore, rather than just work at the same rate of energy utilization with relatively more energy coming from fat and less from carbohydrate utilization, it is possible to work at greater rates, drawing upon the same degree of carbohydrate metabolism in conjunction with this increased fat oxidation. In this way, the same degree of glycogen depletion will be attained and the subjective impressions of fatigue will be the same,

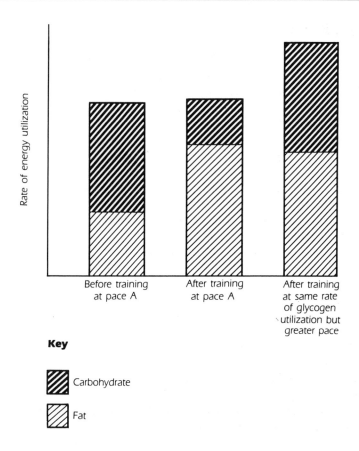

Key

[carbohydrate pattern] Carbohydrate

[fat pattern] Fat

Fig.3.8 The influence of endurance training on metabolic mixture and the rate of energy utilization. An untrained athlete running at pace A will derive the majority of his energy from glycogen. After training, the same athlete will now use relatively more fat while running at the same pace A, thus sparing glycogen. If the athlete continues to run and train to the same degree of effort, a combination of increased fat utilization and a high rate of energy resynthesis from glycogen will allow the runner to sustain a higher rate of energy utilization and therefore run faster.

yet the performance will be markedly enhanced. This is shown diagramatically in Figure 3.8.

While the metabolic and physiological changes produced by interval or sprint training are less well understood, it is generally believed that these also result in lower rates of glycogen utilization for the same amount of work, as well as an enhanced buffering capacity (see page 139).

Preceding diet

The relative amounts of carbohydrate eaten over the days preceding exercise will determine the amount of carbohydrate stored as glycogen in the liver and muscles. Consequently, reduced glycogen stores at the onset of exercise resulting from an inadequate intake of carbohydrate will limit the amount of energy available to the working muscle during exercise. Despite a shift towards fat metabolism as the principal energy source under these conditions, the point at which the availability of glycogen to support the desired rate of ATP resynthesis becomes limiting is reached much earlier, and the ability to perform exercise is then impaired. Conversely, eating large amounts of carbohydrate over several days before performing exercise (as an athlete on a carbohydrate-loading regimen, would do, see page 96) will result in greater than normal stores of glycogen within the liver and muscle and a relatively greater proportion of the total energy supply will come from carbohydrate. There is evidence that this will result in an increased endurance capacity in terms of duration, but whether elevated glycogen stores can lead to improvements in performance through an increased rate of work is less clear. This important point is discussed in detail in Chapter 4.

Ketogenic diet

The shift towards fat metabolism can be enhanced further by totally eradicating carbohydrate from the diet. There is some laboratory evidence that eating a diet that is adequate in all respects apart from carbohydrate (ie, high-energy, high-protein and fat yet very low in carbohydrate — often called a ketogenic diet as it causes an increase in ketone byproducts) for several weeks or months results in changes leading to an increased capacity to utilize fats and ketones. When the glycogen reserves of the body are depleted in this way, the body is totally dependent upon gluconeogenesis to maintain a constant glucose supply. But this glycogen-sparing effect, achieved forcibly, is not necessarily associated with an impaired endurance capacity. (Similar effects can also be brought about, and more rapidly, by a period of fasting).

There are, however, three points to consider before adopting the ketogenic approach:

- The improvements in performance are in duration rather than rate — so you can go on longer rather than faster.
- The effects on performance have only been observed at relatively low exercise intensities (say, 50–60 per cent $\dot{V}O_2max$), where the rate of energy utilization can be adequately covered by fat metabolism and

gluconeogenesis without any appreciable demands on glycogen stores. It is likely that, at higher exercise intensities, the rate of energy resynthesis that can be achieved without the contribution from glycogen would limit performance.

● The lack of carbohydrate in the diet would limit the ability to train, so any metabolic and physiological adaptations produced by exercise would be minimal.

This regimen requires further study and is not to be recommended at the moment.

Caffeine/sugars

A shift towards fat metabolism and glycogen-sparing, with associated improvements in endurance performance, has been reported following consumption of caffeine prior to and during prolonged exercise. In contrast, eating large amounts of simple sugars either immediately before or during exercise can shift the balance in the opposite direction (towards utilizing carbohydrate as an energy source), thus making the body more dependent on its limited glycogen stores rather than sparing glycogen (see Chapter 9).

You always use glycogen

So, no matter what type of exercise you do, how fit you are or what sort of diet you eat, you will always use some glycogen. And, unless the supply of glycogen is maintained, the rate at which energy may be resynthesized, and exercise performed, is limited.

What causes fatigue

Fatigue is another of those words with many meanings in everyday use ranging from a general feeling of tiredness and lethargy to complete and total exhaustion. In strict physiological terms, it can be defined as the inability to maintain the desired rate of work. Exhaustion, in contrast, means the inability to perform work at **any** level.

While the occurrence of fatigue may be readily discernible as a reduction in running speed, it may also manifest itself in many less obvious ways. For example, in a field sport, fatigue could result in an inability to sprint to the ball despite being able to continue running at a pace sufficient to keep up with play, or, on reaching the ball, being unable to bring about the finer motor skills required to control or accurately strike it. Similarly, the dropped

65

catch, the inability to maintain form, or even the lack of concentration over the latter stages of competition, are all subtle reflections of fatigue that can seriously impair performance in a competitive sporting situation.

One of the simplest way of viewing fatigue is as a mismatch of the rates of energy utilization and resynthesis (see page 36). An energy crisis can result when the rate of energy resynthesis cannot keep pace with the demands of energy utilization. This imbalance in resynthesis and utilization must be corrected in order to prevent the concentration of ATP within the cell falling markedly. The simplest way of achieving this is to reduce the rate at which energy is used: how this is done depends on the nature of the exercise task.

Prolonged endurance exercise

One of the principal factors limiting the rate of energy resynthesis is the availability of substrate to meet the demands of energy utilization and, in particular, the contribution made by glycogen within the muscle to the total rate of ATP resynthesis.

The situation of the marathon runner illustrates this (see Figure 3.9):

- Over the first 5–10 miles, the rate of energy utilization may be met by combusting a mixture of carbohydrate and fat as fuel. The contribution made by intramuscular glycogen stores may represent some 45–50 per cent of the total rate of energy resynthesis, the remainder coming from glucose and fatty acids.
- As the stores of glycogen become depleted, the relative contribution made by fatty acids and glucose oxidation increases and, over the middle sections of the race, the rate at which energy is required can be maintained through this increased supply.
- Over the latter stages, however, the reduced contribution from glycogen metabolism reduces the rate at which energy may be resynthesized. Despite increasing rates of energy provision from fat and glucose oxidation, the necessary rate of energy resynthesis still cannot keep pace with the rate at which energy is being used. This mismatch of energy usage and production may well be perceived by the runner as increasing difficulty in maintaining the desired pace.

The only way of correcting this energy deficit is to reduce the rate at which energy is being used so that the rate of energy provision can once again keep pace. This is simply achieved by reducing the running speed: once the rate at which energy is being used is back within the capacity of the muscle to generate energy, it is possible to continue working.

If the runner ignores the signals, a more dramatic form of fatigue may

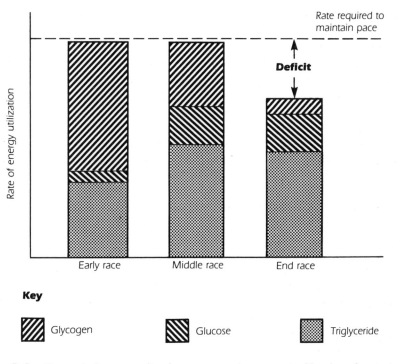

Fig.3.9 The relative contributions to total energy utilization from the oxidation of triglyceride (as intramuscular triglyceride and free fatty acids), glucose and glycogen over various stages of a marathon. By the middle of the race, there is a shift to greater triglyceride and glucose oxidation as the glycogen stores diminish. If the contribution made by depleted glycogen reserves falls by too much, the rate of energy resynthesis from triglyceride and glucose oxidation will be insufficient to match the rate of energy utilization; in this circumstance the runner must run at a slower pace.

occur. It may be possible to continue working in some fashion through making up the energy deficit by altering gait or running style. This would recruit different muscle fibres within the same muscle or different muscle groups, but cannot be continued indefinitely. Eventually the extent of the deficit will become so great that the runner is forced to stop completely or to walk; if the pace had been reduced slightly to keep in line with the capacity to generate energy, the runner could still be running. This lack of pace judgement and failure to respond to the signals of the body results in attempts to 'run through the energy deficit'. This may explain why some marathon runners 'hit the wall' while others deny its very existence.

Pace judgement

It is important to remember that the muscle does not have to be totally depleted of glycogen before the lack of suitable substrate may impair performance. Several studies have shown that, during running at around 70–80 per cent $\dot{V}O_2$max, the rate of glycogen depletion is greatest in the more oxidative SO fibres (see Figure 3.10A). This would suggest that, at this level of effort, it is these fibres that are primarily responsible for generating the tension within the working muscle. As exercise proceeds, the number of SO fibres containing stores of glycogen adequate to maintain the desired rate of energy resynthesis diminishes and they are no longer recruited. Consequently, increasing numbers of the more glycolytic FOG and FG fibres are recruited — until they too become depleted. In this way, more and more of these fibres will become progressively fatigued and be unable to contribute to the generation of tension necessary to maintain the desired running speed.

This would explain why, during endurance exercise, the apparent effort required to maintain the same pace is so much greater over the last few miles compared with the first miles which is why so many endurance athletes slow down over the latter stages of a race. Pace judgement is therefore crucial: ideally, the pace would be such that your glycogen stores expired just as you crossed the finish!

Maximal exercise

In the same way that there is a selective fatigue of the SO fibres during prolonged endurance exercise, during maximal exercise the number of fibres that may be recruited may also be reduced as fatigue occurs. There is evidence, for example, that the more glycolytic FG fibres are more rapidly depleted of glycogen, accumulate more lactate and exhibit greater acidity at exhaustion than the SO fibres, during maximal exercise (see Figure 3.10B). The SO fibres may remain fully operational, but they cannot generate the required tension for the body to continue working at the desired rate. So, during maximal work, fatigue may develop as the number of FG fibres available to generate the tension necessary decreases.

Yet in contrast to prolonged low-intensity exercise, fatigue during maximal exercise (such as sprinting or power events) is not simply just the result of diminishing energy reserves being unable to meet the demands for energy. Rather it may almost be viewed as a response designed to protect the body from self-destruction.

During truly maximal exercise, energy is used at a very high rate — at least three times greater than that required during endurance exercise. This level of demand can only be met by maximal rates of lactate formation and CP utilization. Working indefinitely with such an elevated energy turnover would result in a rapid depletion of CP, maximal accumulation of lactate and

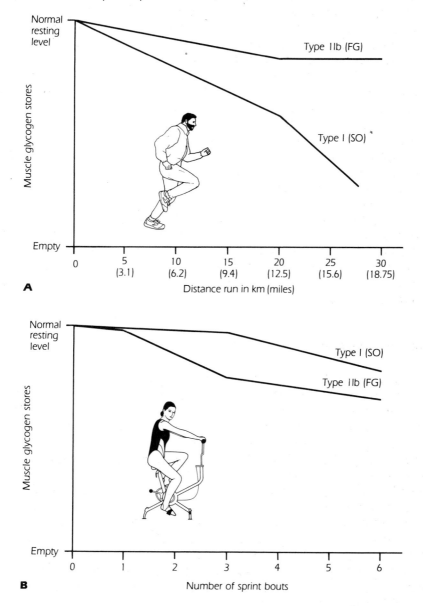

Fig.3.10 Rates of muscle glycogen depletion in different types of skeletal muscle fibre, (a) during prolonged exercise and (b) during repeated sprints.

hydrogen ions and, with decreasing contributions from these processes to the production of energy, a very rapid fall in ATP within the cells. It is estimated that the formation of hydrogen ions would be so rapid that, before the glycogen reserves were totally depleted, the amount of acid within the body would have increased so dramatically as to be fatal!

To prevent total self destruction, the body then needs a way of slowing the rates of glycogen utilization, CP depletion and hydrogen ion accumulation. It must, at the same time, lower the rate at which energy is being used: if energy production slowed, with energy consumption carrying on as before, it would be disastrous.

Hydrogen ion accumulation

These important requirements make the belief that the accumulation of hydrogen ions within the muscle (from the production of lactate) could limit both the production and the utilization of energy particularly appealing. There is in fact considerable evidence that this end-product of energy production could slow down the synthesis of more ATP (and hence of itself) by inhibiting the activites of the enzymes in the energy-producing pathways. Similarly, it has been demonstrated that this accumulation of hydrogen ions may limit the capacity to form cross-bridges between actin and myosin (see page 50) and therefore reduce the rate at which energy is used. This would show itself as a reduced ability to generate force or the inability of the limbs to continue through the intended range of motion (for example, the legs buckling during the latter stages of a 400 metre race). The subjective feelings of pain and discomfort will also reduce the willingness of the athlete to continue working and may in themselves force the individual to stop exercising completely.

Fatigue during team games and field sports

The previous examples were rather extreme forms of exercise. In reality, the majority of sports are intermittent activities — in varying proportions — of endurance exercise and bursts of intense sprint-like activity. So the fatigue processes that limit performance during endurance and maximal activities may both be operational during intermittent activities. In field games (such as soccer, rugby, American football, hockey), canoeing or combat sports, for example, fatigue may be the result of both substrate depletion and lactic acid accumulation affecting energy resynthesis and utilization. Also, while glycogen stores are rarely completely depleted during prolonged endurance activity (as some glycogen would remain in the relatively unrecruited FG fibres), it may be possible to deplete fully all muscle fibres of glycogen during a particularly prolonged period of intermittent exercise because all types of fibre would be recruited.

Summary

■ There are three main types of muscle fibre: Type I fibre (slow oxidative) and the two Type II fibres — Type IIa (fast oxidative glycolytic fibre) and Type IIb (fast glycolytic fibre).

■ The contraction of the muscle fibre, and therefore muscular movement, is the result of an interaction between the two contractile proteins (actin and myosin) and requires energy in the form of ATP.

■ At rest, the rate of ATP utilization is relatively slow, so sufficient ATP can be resynthesized from the oxidation of fats, requiring little carbohydrate. When the rate of energy utilization increases during exercise, the rate of energy resynthesis must also increase.

■ At the onset of exercise and during maximal exercise, the rate of fat oxidation is insufficient to keep pace with the rate of ATP utilization, so energy is derived primarily from CP degradation and lactate formation.

■ Once a steady-state condition has been reached, there is a shift towards the oxidation of intramuscular stores of glycogen and triglyceride as well as blood-borne supplies of free fatty acids (from adipocytes) and glucose (from the liver). Then as these stores become limited, the muscle cell is increasingly dependent upon free fatty acids and glucose delivered by the blood. Liver glycogen stores also fall, so the output of glucose from the liver is derived mainly from gluconeogenesis.

■ If the rate of ATP resynthesis cannot match the rate of utilization, the athlete must reduce his rate of exercise to prevent fatigue.

- The relative utilization of fuel by the muscle during exercise (the metabolic mixture) is dictated by the intensity and duration of the task, the training status of the individual, and the preceding diet.

- No matter what exercise you do, or how fit you are, you will always use some glycogen, so the rate at which exercise can be performed is limited to your supply of glycogen. The harder, longer and more frequently you exercise, the greater the amount of glycogen you will use and the more dependent you will become on ensuring adequate supplies of carbohydrate.

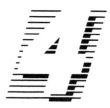

Nutrition and training

Why you should eat more carbohydrate

Carbohydrate and performance

One of the first studies demonstrating that carbohydrate in the diet is important in determining performance during exercise was conducted by Scandinavian researchers over fifty years ago. Subjects were asked to ride a cycle ergometer (a stationary cycle designed to measure muscular work in the laboratory) at a constant exercise intensity (around 70 per cent $\dot{V}O_2$max). After consuming a normal diet they were able to exercise for about two hours before they were exhausted but after eating a diet containing large amounts of carbohydrate for several days before exercising, they were able to continue for nearly twice as long. In contrast, following several days of a diet with very little carbohydrate, performance was impaired — subjects could only exercise for 60–90 minutes. Endurance performance appears, then, to be related to how much carbohydrate there is in the diet.

The energy stores of the body provide the link between diet and performance. No matter what type of exercise, your body needs energy — the harder you exercise, the more energy you need. The muscles doing the work during exercise get much of their energy from the glycogen stores within the muscles and the liver.

Unfortunately, the body's stores of carbohydrate are not that great (600–800 kcal/2500–3400 kJ) about the same amount of carbohydrates that you get each day from the food you eat. If, when running at marathon pace, you were able to use only carbohydrates as a source of energy, these stores would last for 70–80 minutes. When the stores of muscle glycogen are depleted, the ability to perform exercise is severely limited.

However, your muscles can also get energy from a much greater store — free fatty acids released from the fat depots stored beneath the skin. So, by using a mixture of both carbohydrate and fat as fuel, the body can make these limited carbohydrate reserves last considerably longer. It is worth noting that endurance training conditions the body to use proportionately more fat as fuel during exercise — so it can be thought of as glycogen-sparing.

Whenever you exercise, your body tries to ensure that the rate energy is used is matched by the rate it is being produced:

- At relatively low exercise intensities, such as a slow steady jog, the required rate of energy provision is achieved by burning a mixture of carbohydrates and fat. Some carbohydrate must be used, as the body simply cannot produce energy fast enough by burning only fat.
- When exercising maximally, the energy requirement is so great, and needed so quickly, that only carbohydrates can produce energy fast enough, and very little fat is used. So the harder you exercise, the greater the rate at which you use up your glycogen stores.

Maintaining glycogen reserves

You must remember that, whatever exercise is performed, some carbohydrate will always be used. The longer or harder the exercise, the greater the demands placed upon the carbohydrate stores of the body. One of the primary limitations to maintaining high rates of energy expenditure is the availability of glycogen to keep up the desired rate of ATP resynthesis, so the only way to redress an imbalance in energy supply and demand is to decrease the requirement for ATP (ie, slowing down the rate at which work is performed).

The necessity of maintaining glycogen reserves is probably less obvious during training than during competition. Every time an athlete trains, the amount of glycogen within the working muscle falls. As these stores are limited, they must be adequately repleted, or the next training session will be started with lower than normal glycogen reserves. The point at which glycogen becomes limiting will then be attained more rapidly, reducing both the quality and the quantity of training accomplished.

The two principal factors limiting the rate at which glycogen is repleted within skeletal muscle are time and the availability of suitable substrate. Complete repletion of muscle glycogen reserves after prolonged exercise which has totally depleted muscle glycogen may take forty-eight hours or more — irrespective of the intake of carbohydrate over that period (see Figure 4.1). Also, it appears that the trauma associated with heavy training sessions (such as speedwork, gymnasium/weights work and hill running or competition) results in even longer delays in restoring normal muscle glycogen levels. The cellular damage inflicted on the muscle by extreme effort appears to impair the process of glycogen resynthesis and it may take seven days or more to refuel fully after the rigours of a marathon, no matter what the carbohydrate intake.

It should be noted that glycogen stores will remain low **UNLESS** carbohydrate is consumed.

As the body has only a limited capacity to make carbohydrate from substrates other than carbohydrate (eg protein), the body is dependent on the sugars and starches in the diet to replete glycogen.

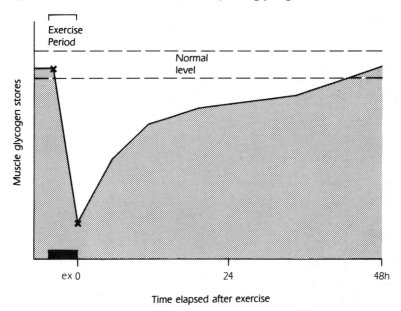

Fig.4.1 Changes in muscle glycogen stores following exercise. Note that complete repletion takes 24–48 hours.

High-carbohydrate diet helps glycogen refuelling

So one of the greatest problems facing the athlete is achieving adequate glycogen repletion to maintain normal energy reserves. This clearly requires time but it has recently been shown that, after exercise-induced glycogen depletion, a diet high in carbohydrate will actually increase the rate of refuelling.

A recent study measured the amount of glycogen in the muscle in three groups of men before and after performing a heavy training session. On completion of a 10 mile (16 km) run followed by some interval running, glycogen stores in the muscles of the legs had decreased by about 60–70 per cent. Each group was then placed on a diet containing different amounts of carbohydrate: 375 g/13 oz, 525 g/19 oz or 650 g/23 oz of carbohydrate per day. Twenty-four hours later, the amount of glycogen in the muscles was remeasured: the two groups consuming 525 g/19 oz per day or more had effectively refuelled, but the group consuming only 375 g/13 oz per day only partially refilled their glycogen reserves (see Figure 4.2).

75

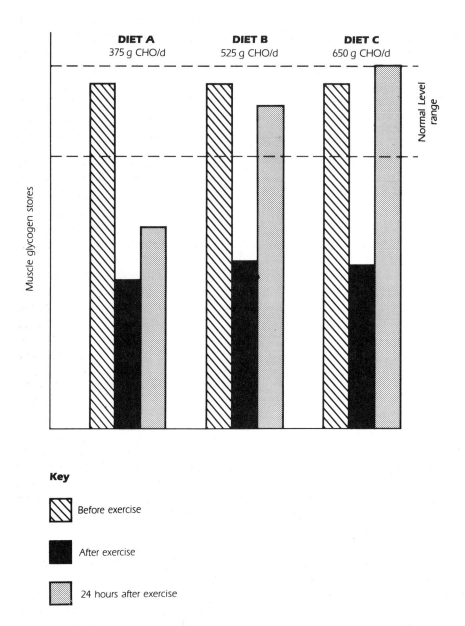

DIET A
375 g CHO/d

DIET B
525 g CHO/d

DIET C
650 g CHO/d

Normal Level range

Muscle glycogen stores

Key

Before exercise

After exercise

24 hours after exercise

Fig.4.2 The effect of different amounts of carbohydrate in the diet on the refuelling of muscle glycogen in the 24–48 hours following exercise. The higher the amount of carbohydrate in the diet, the faster the muscle glycogen stores are replenished.

What should be noted here is that most male athletes in Western countries would probably consume around 250–400 g/9–14 oz of carbohydrate per day as the average intake of male adults within the general population. This would suggest that many athletes are failing to refuel their body stores of carbohydrate sufficiently within twenty-four hours.

It is not simply a case of eating more energy in terms of calories, but the right type of energy — the amount of carbohydrate in the diet is what is important. And a diet containing more than 500 g/18 oz of carbohydrate each day is clearly a high (or very high) carbohydrate diet.

Repeat this inadequate refuelling process over several days and your glycogen stores will be so low that even the lightest exercise becomes extremely difficult to complete. Studies in the early 1970s clearly demonstrated that running 10 miles (16 km) a day for three consecutive days on a diet containing around 350 g/12 oz of carbohydrate per day resulted in a progressive depletion of muscle glycogen with a very low level indeed after the third run (see Figure 4.3).

How many athletes are familiar with that 'end of the week' feeling, staleness, continual lethargy, heavy tired muscles, incomplete recovery between training sessions and the overtraining phenomenon? These may all be related to attempting to train with insufficient repletion of muscle glycogen. Taking concentrated vitamin or mineral supplements will do little to shake off this feeling of being 'run down' or 'stale' — attention should be directed first towards the diet in general and carbohydrates in particular.

Help is at hand, however. The previous study was repeated, with the obvious modification. If a high carbohydrate diet speeds the refuelling process, would eating more carbohydrate lead to a better maintainance of glycogen stores over the period? It was found that a diet containing about 500 g/18 oz of carbohydrate per day reduced the progressive glycogen depletion rate by allowing more glycogen to be repleted between each run (see Figure 4.3). Even though it was not possible to refuel completely between runs, on completion of the study the glycogen stores were much greater than when only 350 g/12 oz of carbohydrate was consumed:

These results highlight three key points:

- A diet rich in carbohydrate will help ensure that your limited reserves of glycogen are refilled between training sessions.
- Variety in training is important so that you have days of heavy glycogen depletion interspersed with days where glycogen stores are not so heavily taxed.
- A rest day is important — resist the temptation to train every day. With no activity, little glycogen is used and the free time can be devoted to preparing plenty of carbohydrate-rich foods for the next few days.

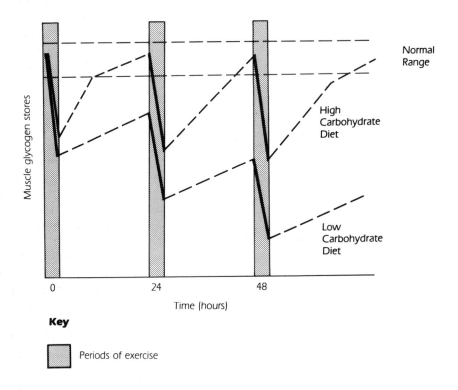

Muscle glycogen stores

Normal Range

High Carbohydrate Diet

Low Carbohydrate Diet

0   24   48

Time (hours)

Key

Periods of exercise

Fig.4.3 The effect of different amounts of carbohydrate in the diet on the refuelling of muscle glycogen following three bouts of exercise within a 72-hour period. There is a significant difference between the rate of refuelling on a high carbohydrate diet and one that is insufficient in carbohydrate.

The refuelling process should start as soon as possible after a training session. Ironically the ability of muscle to replete glycogen is greatest in the first hour following exercise — just the time when you probably feel least like eating. So, rather than wait you should make sure that some carbohydrate is available within an hour. This is particularly important if you are training most days or twice a day.

Deciding what foods to eat

So what should you eat? Clearly, those foods rich in carbohydrate — but especially starchy foods rich in unrefined complex carbohydrate. These include: whole grain cereals and cereal products (wholemeal or whole wheat bread, granola or muesli etc), fresh or dried fruit, fresh or frozen vegetables (particularly root vegetables), beans, peas and lentils. Not only are these high-fibre foods high in carbohydrate, but also in fibre, protein, vitamins and minerals. So simply paying attention to the carbohydrate sources in your diet will also increase substantially your intake of many other valuable nutrients.

Eating for performance and for health

The exact relationship between glycogen repletion and the amount, type and frequency of carbohydrate consumption has not yet been established, but it is generally agreed that the diet should be high in carbohydrates (approximately 50–60 per cent of the total energy intake or more than 500 g/ 18 oz for adult male athletes with a high energy expenditure), with a corresponding reduction in total fat and protein intake. As this is essentially the same advice on healthy eating that is being given to all members of the population (see Chapter 1), there is no conflict between eating for performance and eating for health. Moreover an interest in sport may help introduce healthy eating to an otherwise apathetic audience — the young adolescent, in particular.

Certainly it would appear that the majority of athletes have the same sort of diet as most non-athletes — often unbalanced, unhealthy and insufficiently rich in carbohydrate. This is partly due to lack of knowledge, but may also be explained by the practical constraints of the athlete's lifestyle. These are obviously specific to each individual and should be taken into consideration before offering advice — a single standardized set of dietary guidelines almost invariably results in poor compliance. For example, one of the greatest difficulties facing the athlete is simply fitting in the purchase, preparation and consumption of relatively large amounts of food with the time demands of training, travel, competition and employment or education. Also, eating a high-carbohydrate diet, using mainly starchy, high-fibre foods, is a problem in itself, given the sheer bulk of food that must be consumed for the same amount of carbohydrate found in foods containing simple sugars.

All too often athletes, to satisfy their appetite, rely heavily on foods high in simple carbohydrates in a concentrated form, such as confectionery, preserves, 'junk foods' and sugar itself. Alternatively, they take advantage of the convenience of fast foods — either purchased away from home or prepared simply from the freezer — to save time. Even worse, many athletes find they have to fit their eating around their training schedule and so tend to limit their diet to foods that can be eaten and tolerated just before training. These foods are often low in complex carbohydrates and lacking in many other nutrients, yet high in sugar and fat.

79

Junking the 'junk foods'?

One cautionary point, however. The current dietary advice to the general public is to reduce their intake of simple sugars but whether this is less applicable to athletes in regular training has yet to be established. It appears to be the excessive sugar intake that is undesirable in health terms — the excess energy is stored as triglyceride and may be a major contributory factor in the development of many Western diseases. In athletes, however, carbohydrate intake over and above requirements is less likely to be a problem. More often than not the reverse is the case.

Yet, before totally excluding simple carbohydrate ('junk') foods from the diet, remember that they provide a large proportion of the total carbohydrate. Eliminating them completely could result in as much as a 50–80 per cent reduction in the carbohydrate intake of some athletes — particularly the young. If you remove such foods from your usual diet in order to improve its overall quality, alternative sources of carbohydrate of comparable density must be included to stop total carbohydrate intake falling considerably. For example, you could substitute granola or muesli bars for confectionery, and pizzas for hamburgers.

What type of carbohydrate?

The relative merits of one form of carbohydrate over another, and the number and timing of meals, in promoting the repletion of muscle glycogen is still the focus of much research. It appears, however, that complex and simple carbohydrates are equally effective in glycogen repletion. Certainly, both are required in the diet to achieve very high intakes of carbohydrate. But the added benefits of an increased consumption of fibre, vitamins and minerals, with an accompanying decrease in fat intake comes with the choice of carbohydrates. Eating large amounts of fat takes up calories that would be more energy-effective if devoted to complex carbohydrates.

How much carbohydrate?

Exactly how much carbohydrate **you** should eat cannot be determined simply. Consuming 500 g/18 oz of carbohydrate per day or more is easily possible if you have a high energy diet providing around 4000 kcal/16.7 MJ per day (so that around 50 per cent of the total energy intake comes from carbohydrate). Yet, as 500 g/18 oz of carbohydrate alone provides around 2000 kcal/8.3 MJ, this carbohydrate intake would be impossible to achieve on a relatively low-energy diet. Getting 50 per cent of total energy from carbohydrate in a diet providing only 1000 kcal/4.2 MJ would involve a carbohydrate intake of only 125 g/4 oz. Even if **all** the energy came from carbohydrate, it would still represent only around 250 g/9 oz and would be extremely unbalanced!

Such low intakes of energy are frequently reported, though not every athlete consumes more than 3000 kcal/12.5 MJ per day, as is often supposed. Those participating in competitions where strict weight categories are enforced (such as lightweight combat sports, rowing) often habitually consume less than 1500 kcal/6.3 MJ. Similarly, young female distance runners, gymnasts and ballet dancers, as well as professional jockeys, often intentionally restrict their food intake to maintain low body weight. So low carbohydrate intakes are another problem associated with low energy intakes (see Figure 4.4). But, as many lightweight athletes — particularly females — tend to be smaller, their requirement for carbohydrate to refuel their smaller muscles should be less, so it is unlikely that they would require more than 500 g/18 oz of carbohydrate per day.

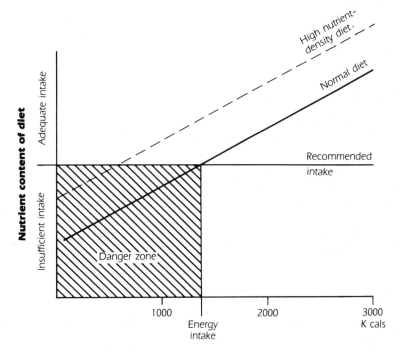

Fig.4.4 The amount of food eaten each day is linearly related to the daily energy intake ie, the greater the amount of food eaten, the greater the intake of nutrients. When inadequate amounts of food are consumed as when restricting energy intake, the nutrient content of the diet may fail to meet the requirements of the body; the lower the energy intake, the greater the need to consume foods rich in essential nutrients to avoid malnourishment.

In accordance with current advice on healthy eating, carbohydrates ideally should provide half or more of the total energy in the diet. Rather than trying to prescribe a fixed amount of carbohydrate for yourself, the best approach is to concentrate on carbohydrate-rich foods at most meals and avoid eating habits that intentionally limit carbohydrate intake.

But be careful that eating more carbohydrate does not make your total energy intake shoot up. If the total amount of fat in the diet is not reduced, the excess energy will be stored and you will put on weight!

Making a meal of it

What does all this mean in practical teams?
1. Start the day with a high-carbohydrate breakfast — such as home-made granola or muesli, wholemeal or whole wheat toast and fresh fruit juice.
2. If breakfast is missed because of training, make sure that some carbohydrate-rich foods are eaten mid-morning — granola or muesli bars are useful between meals.
3. Lunch could consist of sandwiches made using whole grain bread with a low-fat filling, and fresh fruit.
4. If you are training in the early evening before the main meal of the day, why not have a mid-afternoon snack? This will prevent those weak and dizzy sensations, normally associated with hunger, as you train.
5. For your evening meal, resist the temptation to have large portions of meat and concentrate on the vegetables instead. The humble potato, cooked in its skin and with a variety of possible fillings, is ideal. Alternatively, whole grain rice, pastas, cracked wheat or oats are staple foods that can form the basis for many different meals. And you can always use more legumes or pulses in side dishes as a change from traditional vegetables.

Adopting a new approach

Fitting this new approach towards food into your present lifestyle may be difficult. Training and other commitments may often leave you little time to think about what food to eat, let alone purchase and prepare. But persevere, the rewards are worth it, not just in terms of performance but, just as importantly, for the sake of your health!

A good diet may make its greatest impact on your performance simply by helping you to recover more effectively between training sessions. As improvements in performance are primarily the result of how well your body adapts to the stimulus of intensive and, above all, **consistent** training, it is important that the supply of carbohydrate is maintained to sustain glycogen reserves throughout. Without adequate energy reserves within the muscle, you will not be able to train to your full potential and, without training, there will be only minor improvements in performance. So it is vitally important to pay attention to eating habits throughout the year — not just in those days of competition.

Recommendations: your basic training diet

■ Good nutrition can make its greatest impact by helping you to recover between training sessions. Improvements in performance are primarily the result of your body's adaptation to the stresses of intensive training. With **consistent** training comes adaptation, with adaptation comes improvement. So it is important that you pay attention to your eating habits 365 days of the year — not just on those days of competition.

■ One of the prime considerations is that your diet meets the demands placed upon your body by training. In particular, you must consume sufficient energy in the form of carbohydrates to maintain the stores of energy within the muscles. Low carbohydrate intakes while you are training hard can only result in low muscle glycogen stores. Training on low glycogen stores is hard.

■ Start the refuelling process as soon as you can after you finish training. You have only a limited time available to consume a relatively large amount of food. The muscles' capacity to refuel is greatest over that first hour after training.

■ Organize yourself. Remember that you **must** refuel, so don't compromise. Fit your eating around your training. If you miss breakfast to train, have a high-carbohydrate mid-morning snack (granola or muesli bars, etc). If you train in the evening, eat something around 3–4 in the afternoon and have your main meal **after** training. Your appetite will probably increase as the volume and intensity of training increases, so eat more carbohydrates but don't overeat.

■ Don't restrict your eating to traditional mealtimes — you may end up gorging on just three meals a day. Try taking smaller but more frequent meals, plus several snacks.

83

■ At least one rest day a week is important — give your body time to recover from the stresses of training. Use the extra time to eat sensibly and make up for any hurried meals eaten during training. Above all, refuel your carbohydrate stores. It is probably better to work on a three-day training programme, then rest for one day, than train for six days before having a day off.

■ Eat more fresh or frozen vegetables (particularly root and green leafy vegetables), potatoes, fresh and dried fruit (particularly citrus fruits), cereals, (whole wheat pasta, brown rice, granola or muesli, etc), nuts, beans and legumes (peas, all types of beans, lentils, etc). All these foods are high in carbohydrate, fibre, vitamins and minerals — in one tasty package — while being relatively low in energy. They're only fattening when you **add** large amounts of fat.

■ Place the emphasis on starchy rather than sugary foods when attempting to increase your carbohydrate intake — do not rely solely on confectionery or sweet foods to provide you with carbohydrate.

■ Increase your bread consumption (preferably wholemeal, whole-wheat, or granary) but take care not to layer it with fat. If making sandwiches with a moist filling, reduce the amount of butter or margarine.

■ There is no need to eat large amounts of red meat. Select leaner cuts of meat or try using white meats such as chicken or turkey. Alternatively, reduce your overall meat consumption and fill up on high-carbohydrate foods. Try eating at least one meat-free meal each day or construct meals that use a little meat sparingly throughout the dish (paella, risotto, pasta dishes, Chinese-style cooking).

■ Reduce your consumption of meat products (beefburgers, sausages, spreads, etc), pies and pastries — these can all contain large amounts of fat.

■ Reduce your consumption of fried foods – try broiling or grilling, stir-frying or steaming instead. Pour off any fat that appears during cooking. Try not to add excessive amounts of fat to a dish (gravy, sauces, butter on hot toast or baked potatoes).

■ Try alternatives to mayonnaise or oil-based dressings for salads — natural yogurt or citrus fruit juice can be used on their own or as the basis for less oily dressings.

■ Invest in a wok and 'flash-fry' foods at a very high heat with minimal fat or oil. This type of cooking seals the food rapidly and helps to retain its nutrients.

■ Alternatively, try to gain access to a microwave cooker. Microwave cooking food does not cause any appreciable losses in nutrients yet can save considerable amounts of time — something vital to the busy athlete. Rather than simply heat commercial pre-prepared meals, make your own meals during the quieter periods of the week or rest days, store in the freezer and re-heat as required.

■ Ensure that you maintain a high-fluid intake by drinking plenty of water and fresh fruit juice (high in minerals) as part of your normal diet. Ensure that you are never dehydrated before or during **any** training session (see Chapter 5). Organize your training so that you can take small amounts of fluid regularly. Be careful of alcohol — don't try to train on a hangover.

■ Take a positive interest in your food. Don't simply eat what is put in front of you. Take care in planning meals and choosing and preparing food, even if this means learning to cook for yourself. Above all, enjoy your food — don't become fanatical or obsessed with your training diet.

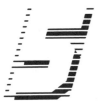

Fluid and the athlete

Temperature regulation during exercise

Man is very inefficient when it comes to converting the energy stored in food into mechanical work: only about 20–25 per cent of the available energy stored in carbohydrate or fat is actually converted into a form that the muscles can use to contract and generate force. The remaining 70–80 per cent of the energy is released as heat. During exercise, when the rate of energy utilization rises, the rate of heat production also increases. So, in order to prevent an excessive rise in body temperature (called **hyper**thermia), the body must take steps to dispose of this additional heat.

The body can lose heat by a variety of mechanisms. It may be gained or lost by any combination of radiation, convection or conduction, depending on the relative temperatures of the body and the environment surrounding it (see Figure 5.1). These processes are generally adequate to cope with heat production when the body is at rest and allow us to maintain a constant body temperature of around 37–38°C/98–100°F. When the rate of heat production increases (during exercise, for example) these avenues of heat loss are inadequate to cope with the rise in heat production unless the temperature of the air surrounding the body is low.

Sweating

As heat production increases, the body calls upon a fourth mechanism — sweating. The evaporation of sweat secreted on to the surface of the skin is a very effective way of losing heat — for every 1 litre/1.75 pints of sweat that evaporates, some 600 kcal/2500 kJ of heat energy may be released from the body. As it is possible to lose as much as 2 litres/3.5 pints of sweat per hour during prolonged exercise in a hot environment, there is appreciable potential for heat loss by this mechanism. However, not all of the sweat formed during exercise is effective in dissipating heat as some does not evaporate on the skin surface but drops off the skin and so does not aid heat loss. This can even be a disadvantage to the heavy sweater.

Although sweating is a very effective way of losing heat, care must be

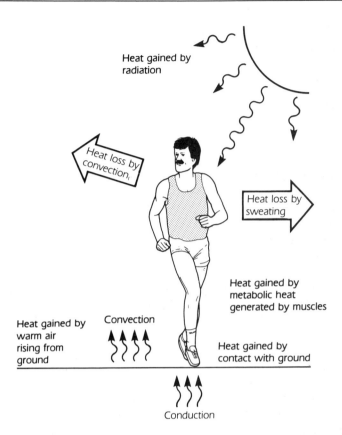

Heat gained by
radiation

Heat loss by
convection

Heat loss by
sweating

Heat gained by
metabolic heat
generated by muscles

Heat gained by
warm air
rising from
ground

Convection

Heat gained by
contact with ground

Conduction

Fig.5.1. Processes by which heat is either released from the body or gained by the body from the surrounding environment during exercise. Note that this is a two-way process and heat may also be lost from the body by convection, conduction and radiation as well as through evaporation of sweat on the skin.

taken to ensure that dehydration does not impair this process. Sweat is simply a dilute version of blood so, when sweating is prolonged or pronounced, the body loses both water and electrolytes. Electrolytes (salts dissolved in the body's fluid) are lost from the body at a much slower rate than water and this does not present an immediate problem. It does not appear to be necessary to replace these electrolytes during exercise — if anything, the concentration of the major electrolytes in plasma tends to increase.

But the water loss will cause serious problems if no attempts are made to replace the lost fluid. Losses of fluid corresponding to as little as 2 per cent of body weight can seriously impair the capacity to perform muscular work.

87

Most athletes may lose 1–5 per cent of their body weight during prolonged exercise even when the climate is temperate and fluid is regularly taken throughout. Under extreme conditions, when temperature and humidity are high, decreases in body weight of as much as 8–10 per cent have been reported. Most of the weight loss observed during exercise is due to the loss of fluid from the body and results in a reduction in plasma volume and the movement of water between the body's fluid compartments — intracellular and extracellular.

Fluid compartments

The total water content of the average 70 kg/154 lb man is about 23 litres/40 pints. Of this, about two-thirds is located within the body cells (intracellular fluid). The remaining third (extracellular fluid), circulates in the spaces between the cells (interstitial water) and mixes with the fluid of the blood (plasma water) through the capillary walls. Fluid diffuses between the extracellular and intracellular compartments of the body by a process called osmosis: openings in the walls of the membranes of cells allow the continual movement of water molecules in and out of the cell.

During osmosis, water moves to the area where the number of water molecules (or concentration of water) is lowest. This is primarily determined by the number of particles dissolved in the water — the greater number of particles in a given volume of water, the fewer water molecules. So water moves to the area with the largest number of particles in solution (see Figure 5.2).

The majority of particles in solution are derived from electrolytes which, when dissolved in body fluids, break down to yield positively and negatively charged ions. Apart from being essential minerals, they also control the movement of water between the fluid compartments of the body. Sodium (Na^+) and chloride (Cl^-) are the ions primarily responsible for maintaining the water content of the extracellular fluid compartment and are lost in greatest quantities in sweat. If a large amount of Na^+ and Cl^- ions is lost in sweat, the body loses part of its control over the distribution and volume of extracellular water and attempts must be made to redistribute water in order to maintain the original water–ion relationship. A severe depletion of these ions over a prolonged period of time leads to progressive water loss from the extracellular compartment, and therefore from plasma volume. This may be severe enough to lead to circulatory failure.

Fluid balance

The body needs to balance the loss and intake of fluids in order to maintain its capacity to regulate body temperature, just like a car needs cooling fluid in

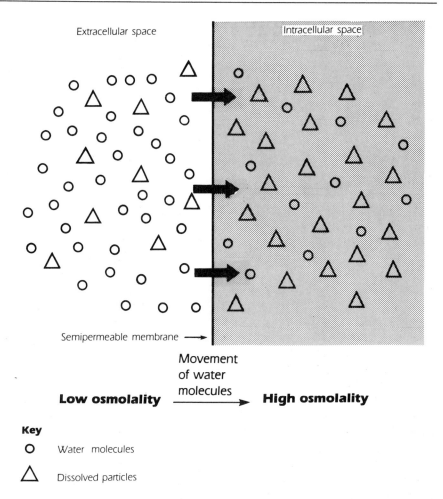

Fig.5.2. Osmosis; the movement of a solvent such as water from a less concentrated to a high concentrated solution across a semipermeable membrane.

the radiator. A reduction in cooling fluid will lead to a reduced ability to remove heat from the engine (the muscles) and deliver it to the radiator (the skin) where heat can be lost. Consequently, the temperature of the system will rise until the engine ceases to work.

Something similar happens in humans when sweat losses greatly exceed replacement:

● The circulatory system is unable to cope and skin blood flow falls. The plasma volume must be preserved in order to maintain the high blood

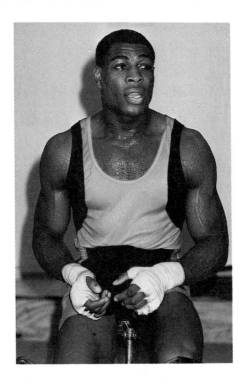

flow both to the working muscle (to deliver oxygen and substrate while removing the end-products of energy metabolism, including heat) and to the skin (in order to sweat freely and dissipate the heat).

- As sweating continues, the water portion of the blood decreases, reducing the volume of blood available to the circulation and making it more difficult to satisfy the energy demands of the muscle and to transfer heat to the environment via the skin.
- As a result of reduced plasma volume, the amount of blood pumped by the heart with each beat (the stroke volume) drops. Heart rate then increases (to maintain cardiac output) and the blood flow to the skin decreases because blood flow to the muscle takes priority.
- A reduction in sweating and in the ability to lose heat accompanies this so, if exercise continues, the temperature of the body climbs steadily from normal towards the danger zone: 41°C/105°F.

In practical terms, performance falls off rapidly at this stage and the effort required to maintain the same exercise intensity increases dramatically — even if the individual does not feel particularly hot. This may ultimately lead to heat exhaustion, with potentially fatal consequences, if action to correct the fluid imbalance and reduce heat production is not taken immediately.

What influences fluid absorption?

Water is mainly absorbed from the intestine, very little in the stomach itself. Once water reaches the intestine, absorption is rapid and relatively unaffected by moderate exercise. So the main limitation to fluid replacement seems to be not **how much** you can drink but **how quickly** the drink can leave the stomach. Many factors have been shown to affect this process (known as the rate of gastric emptying), including how much you drink, its temperature and how hard you are exercising. The relative concentration of any substances, such as carbohydrate or electrolytes, dissolved in the drink will also significantly alter gastric emptying (see page 133).

The importance of gastric emptying

The factors influencing gastric emptying suggest how drinks can best be used by athletes:

- Although larger volumes (up to 600 ml) are emptied from the stomach more rapidly than smaller portions, many athletes find it uncomfortable to exercise on a full stomach and it tends to interfere with breathing — most prefer to drink little and often. Many athletes who become nauseous while exercising have drunk too much fluid which simply sits in the stomach; alternatively, the solution may have been too concentrated – see Chapter 9. How much you should drink will depend on you, what solution you are drinking and how hard you exercise. Everybody is different and the only way to find out is to experiment during training — **do not** wait until competition.
- Colder solutions empty from the stomach more rapidly than warm ones — the ideal temperature appears to be 8–13°C/46–55°F — but do not worry about chilling your stomach: stomach cramps are more likely to be the result of an overconcentrated solution in your stomach than a cold drink.
- The duration of exercise appears to have little effect on the rate of gastric emptying but the intensity is very important. Up to about 75 per cent $\dot{V}O_2$max, the rate of absorption appears unaffected but after that it declines rapidly. So the harder you are working the more difficult it is to replace the fluids lost as you sweat. It has been shown that, at the sort of exercise intensities required to run a 2–10 to 2–20 marathon (that is,

in 2 hours 10–20 minutes), the amount of water that can actually be absorbed is likely to be minimal. This should not be taken to imply that elite athletes do not need to drink!

Do you need to replace the electrolytes lost in sweat during exercise?

Studies have show that, even when a runner loses several litres of sweat, the changes in body electrolytes are minimal. Total body stores of sodium and chloride fall by only 5–7 per cent while magnesium stores are relatively unaltered. As more fluid is lost than electrolytes, the concentration of electrolytes in plasma increases or remains constant.

The athlete is rarely faced with a challenge to the body so severe as to induce electrolyte-associated problems. Although there is some evidence that potassium stores could drop very low after several days of very heavy prolonged exercise, other studies have shown that the body actually conserves sodium and potassium over successive days of heavy sweating. It does this by reducing the excretion of electrolytes in the urine and their secretion in the sweat through the action of a hormone called aldosterone on the kidney and sweat glands. So, as part of the heat acclimatization process, the body adapts to the stress of repeated episodes of dehydration by producing a more abundant yet diluted sweat.

When to take fluids

It is imperative that you train your body to accept fluids whenever you exercise and you should become accustomed to consuming fluid at all exercise intensities, both training and competition. The less well-trained athlete will not be able to sustain a high percentage of their $\dot{V}O_2$max during exercise so he will be able to take in relatively more fluids and carbohydrate into his body. This may be an advantage in endurance sports (for example, a 4–5 hour marathon).

Thirst in itself is a very poor indicator of the need to start taking fluid. By the time the athlete feels thirsty, the losses of fluid during exercise are irreplaceable. So ensuring that the body is fully or overhydrated prior to exercise — **never** dehydrated — and then taking small amounts of fluid little and often from the beginning is of the utmost importance.

Of course, the individual may be aware of the need for fluid consumption during exercise, but the conditions of competition often make it impractical (or, even worse, impossible, because of regulations!) to drink as much as is

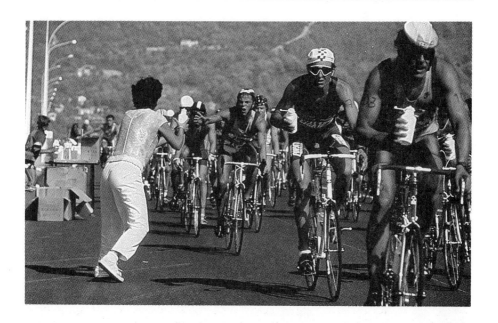

desired. For example, the continuous nature of sports like team games actively prohibits fluid intake during the game itself (40–45 minutes with only informal stoppages), while such activities as the racquet sports have breaks between games or sets. Very few sports, however, have facilities or stoppages which promote fluid intake.

Adequate hydration before, during and after exercise

So considerable care should be taken to ensure adequate hydration before, during and after exercise to avoid thermal distress, and these principles apply equally well to both training and competition. Body water will be progressively depleted over several days of insufficient fluid intake in the same way as glycogen stores are depleted following inadequate carbo-hydrate intake. The feeling of fatigue in the latter stages of prolonged endurance exercise performed in the heat may be as much due to dehydration as to the depletion of energy stores within the muscle. And remember that these points apply to all athletes — not just marathon runners — especially those exercising indoors in warm, humid and enclosed environments (working out in a gym, playing volleyball and basketball, for example).

93

Recommendations: fluid balance

■ You must condition your body to get used to taking fluids by using fluids during training sessions, not just during competition.

■ Make sure that you are always fully hydrated before taking any exercise. Never start exercising in a dehydrated condition. Avoid large amounts of alcohol the night before.

■ Take some fluid prior to exercise, say 250–500 ml of water 20–40 minutes before activity. As urine formation is reduced considerably once you are exercising, the need for an emergency 'pit stop' is unlikely.

■ During exercise, small amounts of fluid should be taken little and often. You should start drinking early on during exercise — do not wait until you are thirsty before drinking. Try using a cyclist's water bottle as a container.

■ Plan for regular water breaks where possible. Athletes should be encouraged to drink even if they are not thirsty.

■ Cold drinks empty from the stomach faster than warm or hot drinks. While larger volumes empty more quickly than smaller volumes, beware of having too much fluid in the stomach!

■ The most important consideration throughout is fluid intake so plain water is the immediate choice. However, when used with care, commercial drinks can assist in the replenishment of fluids while also providing additional carbohydrate to supplement the body's energy reserves. But if used incorrectly they may actually impair performance by causing nausea and stomach discomfort. Worse, they may inhibit fluid absorption and thereby accelerate dehydration. The electrolytes they contain are not present to replace those lost in sweating but to help increase absorption of the fluid (see page 133).

■ Following exercise, start the rehydration process immediately — do not wait for several hours. Ideally, always carry your own supply of fluid in your kit bag so that you are never caught short. Do not rely on the coach or organizer of an event to provide fluid.

■ Salt tablets are to be avoided at all cost. There is ample salt in the diet without having to take extra salt at mealtimes.

■ Splashing water on the skin during exercise will also help you lose heat through evaporation.

■ Acclimatize to exercise in warm environments carefully and adequately prior to competition. Note that young children take longer to acclimatize than mature adults (see page 144).

■ Wear suitable clothing to cope with prevailing climatic conditions.

■ Be aware that as you slow down, the rate of heat production also decreases. While you may have started out in suitable clothing, you may find that too much heat is lost as you tire and your body temperature may fall considerably unless additional clothing is available. **Hypo**thermia (subnormal body temperature) is very common during prolonged endurance competitions (such as the marathon) when people stop running and continue the race at a walk. So always consider how you will finish the exercise task rather than how you feel when you set out.

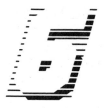

Nutrition and competition

The information in this chapter applies to **all** athletes entering competition. Endurance events such as marathon running are dealt with at length here as most research work has been done in this field.

Preparation for competition

The most important nutritional consideration is ensuring that you start competition fully recovered from the rigours of training with at least **normal** glycogen stores (see page 74). As training will result in substantially lowered glycogen stores, the first step is to reduce the volume of training over the week preceding competition. This, combined with a healthy diet containing adequate amounts of carbohydrate, should ensure that normal glycogen stores are achieved in three to four days. Consumption of a high carbohydrate diet can, however, result in significantly greater than normal glycogen stores: this provides the foundation for a popular dietary manoeuvre called carbohydrate-loading.

What is carbohydrate-loading?

Unlike many nutritional practices favoured by athletes, the carbohydrate-loading regimen does have a scientific basis. Carbohydrate-loading (the consumption of a low-carbohydrate diet for several days after performing prolonged exhaustive exercise, followed by several days of a high-carbohydrate diet), was in fact an important research tool into the factors that limit endurance performance.

Scandinavian research established many years ago the importance of dietary carbohydrate in determining ability to perform prolonged heavy exercise (see page 73).

The carbohydrate-loading regimen was first developed, also in Scandinavia, to determine the relationship between carbohydrate in the diet, the muscle's energy stores and endurance capacity. It was shown that, during heavy prolonged exercise, fatigue was associated with the depletion of the glycogen stores within the exercising muscle but that, if a high-carbohydrate diet was consumed for several days after exhaustive exercise, repletion of the muscle glycogen stores continued beyond the normal pre-exercise levels. This supercompensation of muscle glycogen could then be enhanced still further if a period of carbohydrate restriction was introduced **before** the high carbohydrate diet.

Using the carbohydrate-loading regimen, these researchers were able to show that the ability to perform prolonged exercise on a cycle ergometer was directly related to the size of the initial glycogen stores. Compared to the normal diet condition, exercise time to exhaustion was halved when exercise depletion was followed by carbohydrate restriction, whereas it could be increased by 50 per cent following carbohydrate-loading. Not all the subjects exhibited the same degree of improvement however: the percentage improvement ranged from 1–118 per cent. Therefore, though the carbohydrate-loading regimen appeared to enhance performance, the effect was extremely variable.

Although the duration of work can be extended by carbohydrate-loading, athletic competition demands an increase in the **rate** of work, that is speed! Rather than being able to run for longer, most athletes are concerned with getting to the finish that little bit faster. What evidence is there that carbohydrate-loading actually enhances endurance performance in situations such as a marathon?

Carbohydrate-loading and performance

Apart from the subjective reports by marathoners themselves, there are no reported scientific studies performed over the marathon distance. The only evidence that the regimen is beneficial is from a study performed over 19 miles/30 km; it reported improvements in run time of 1–16 minutes (on average about 6 per cent) after athletes completed the traditional carbohydrate-loading regimen compared with competing after a normal mixed diet. It was found that, although the regimen had little effect on the pace in the early stages of the run, the decrease in pace as fatigue occurred was less pronounced after carbohydrate-loading. This observation fits in well with the view that fatigue during prolonged endurance activity is related to the depletion of muscle glycogen.

For nearly twenty years this experiment has been the only evidence that carbohydrate-loading might improve marathon performance, and no further attempts have been made to extend or even repeat the early work. The results of the studies filtered through to the athletic population, nevertheless. The links between Scandinavian scientists and coaches are strong and their runners were soon using the new diet. It was soon promoted in the USA and the UK and within a few years, 'carbohydrate-loading' was a familiar term in marathon running.

Carbohydrate-loading: the mechanism

Just how does it work? Though the exact mechanism responsible for the glycogen supercompensation effect is not fully understood, there is a logical explanation as to why increasing the amount of energy stored in the muscle should be advantageous.

As discussed earlier, the principal supply of energy during prolonged exercise is derived from both the carbohydrate and fat stores of the body. Carbohydrate is made available from the glycogen stores of the liver and muscle, whilst fat is transported to the muscle in the form of free fatty acids. The relative utilization of carbohydrate or free fatty acids is largely dictated by the energy demand (the energy intensity). Although the energy stored as fat in the body is great, the rate at which ATP can be generated when fat is the predominant fuel, and consequently the exercise intensity it can support, is relatively low. However, at marathon pace (70–85 per cent $\dot{V}O_2max$), ATP is derived principally from glycogen degradation; as these limited stores are gradually depleted by exercise, the only way the muscle can continue providing ATP is by placing progressively increasing demands on free fatty acid oxidation. Unfortunately, the initial rate of ATP supply cannot be sustained and, if the rate of energy supply is less than the rate of energy demand, it becomes increasingly difficult to maintain the same pace.

Avoiding 'the wall'

It is probably this **gradual** mismatch of energy supply in relation to demand that many runners experience as 'the wall': you do not suddenly 'run out of glycogen' and 'switch from glycogen to fat', as is often reported. The subjective feelings of discomfort will certainly be exaggerated in runners who fail to recognize the sensations of fatigue and try to force themselves on at the same pace. Runners who never experience this traumatic event are probably better judges of their pace over the distance and adjust it in relation to their subjective feelings of fatigue.

The effect of carbohydrate-loading is to increase the size of the initial glycogen store. Essentially, if you start with a larger fuel tank, it should last for longer. In other words, carbohydrate-loading places a greater reliance on glycogen as an energy source.

In contrast, the principal adaptation to endurance training is a glycogen-sparing effect. Training effectively allows you to use relatively more fat for a given speed, thus placing less demands upon glycogen. There have recently been several reports of other ways of increasing endurance performance via a glycogen-sparing effect. Training-like effects can be induced in man by caffeine ingestion (see page 138) and in experiments in the rat by fasting or consumption of a carbohydrate-free diet for several weeks. However it should be remembered that man is not a rat! Rats have the distinct advantage of being able to maintain their muscle glycogen stores despite very low carbohydrate intakes. In man, low carbohydrate intakes **always** mean low glycogen levels, which will clearly impair performance. So, until we know more, do not suddenly start experimenting with carbohydrate-free diets, fasting or caffeine over the week before competition!

Can elevated glycogen stores actually be harmful?

There have been some very worrying reports about the potentially harmful effects of carbohydrate-loading. Claims of angina-like pains, electro-cardiogram abnormalities and disruption of skeletal muscle fibres are commonplace — yet these are generally unfounded. The only group particularly at risk are the diabetic runners who should consult their diabetologist before using the regimen.

Most of the alarm has stemmed from the isolated (and misleading) case-history of one runner who gorged as much bread as he could eat for three days as part of a high-carbohydrate diet. He managed to consume two loaves of bread at one meal and then, not surprisingly, complained of abdominal pains. Other problems have been reported in cases of glycogen-storage disease, where the specific enzymes controlling glycogen resynthesis are disturbed. In such conditions, glycogen levels of heart and muscle may increase six to eight fold, rather than the normal two to three fold, after carbohydrate-loading.

Restricting the carbohydrate over the low-carbohydrate phase should, however, be done with caution. It is vital that you keep up your energy intake and only reduce the carbohydrate level during this phase. It is a major mistake to take the regimen to extremes by maintaining heavy training schedules on practically no carbohydrate. After all, the body needs at least 50 g/2 oz of carbohydrate each day just to preserve energy supply to the brain. Over-restriction results in total dependence on fat metabolism and you can easily become ketotic (see page 43). If handled properly, carbohydrate-loading may confer a physiological advantage, rather than be detrimental to health.

Apart from energy supply, the other ever-present problem during exercise is temperature regulation (see page 86) which can only be achieved with adequate fluid maintenance. In storing glycogen you also store water, so dehydration may be **partly** offset by carbohydrate-loading, though never completely, so it is still imperative that you take fluids regularly throughout exercise.

Does carbohydrate-loading work for everybody?

The same variable response shown in the early laboratory studies is also apparent in endurance runners and cyclists. Whether this is because glycogen supercompensation is affected by hereditary factors is uncertain and requires further clarification. There may however be some substance in the belief that well-trained athletes will derive less benefit from carbohydrate-loading than the type of athlete who takes over four hours to complete a marathon distance.

This may be illustrated by the performance study described on page 97. Although all the subjects were physical education students, some were casual runners who did little if any training whereas others were regular competitors in cross-country events (the two types of runner can be clearly identified by the $\dot{V}O_2$max values and finishing times). The well-trained runners covered the marathon distance at a pace of around 6.5 min/mile (4.0 min/km) while the others ran at around 8.5 min/mile (5.3 min/km). The improvements in performance were considerably greater in the less trained than in the trained runners.

This may be explained by the fact that, apart from having better pace judgement, the trained runners would start the race with relatively higher levels of muscle glycogen on the normal diet as a function of training alone. Training would also give a greater capacity to utilize free fatty acids, thereby placing a lesser dependency upon muscle glycogen. Thus the potential benefits of further increases in glycogen levels would be of less value to highly trained runners than to those runners whose glycogen stores may be limiting. This would suggest that the longer you exercise, the more benefit you may find from carbohydrate-loading, but this theoretical conclusion is not supported by any direct evidence.

Eating enough carbohydrate

The debate as to the efficacy of carbohydrate-loading may also be related to the varying degrees of success athletes have had in altering carbohydrate intake. A lack of effect may simply be due to inadequate dietary manipulation. Although eating more carbohydrate seems relatively easy, many people select different foods but fail to increase their carbohydrate intake substantially. In a simple study conducted on carbohydrate-loading, it was found that many subjects found it easy to restrict their carbohydrate intake over the low-carbohydrate phase of the carbohydrate-loading regimen, but relatively few were able to increase their carbohydrate intake by more than 40 per cent over that consumed on their normal diet. Lack of knowledge resulted not only in insufficient carbohydrate consumption but also large swings in energy intake. The subjects tended to stop eating altogether over the low-carbohydrate phase and then gorge themselves over the high-carbohydrate phase. Over-restriction of carbohydrate during the depletion phase combined with inadequate carbohydrate intake over the loading phase could easily result in lower than normal muscle glycogen levels. If you do decide to follow the traditional carbohydrate-loading regimen, make sure that you plan your food selection carefully — do not leave anything to chance. If it works for you then stick with it. If it hasn't worked before, perhaps you should take a closer look at your diet.

There is little evidence that elevated glycogen stores will improve performance in every sport, but some sports may benefit from increasing the stores of glycogen prior to competition. In tournament situations, for example, when the competition is spread over several days — heats, semifinals and finals in athletics and tennis or playing extra time in field sports such as football — you will get to the finals in a better condition if you start off with a higher glycogen store as this will help to slow down the progressive depletion of glycogen with each bout of the competition.

It should also be noted that the storage of glycogen (plus associated water) is likely to result in increases in body weight — possibly by as much as 2 kg. This may cause problems if competing in specific weight categories (see page 115).

An alternative method of preparing for competition

One of the main disadvantages of trying to follow the traditional carbohydrate-loading regimen is the difficult period of carbohydrate restriction. Many athletes find that combining heavy training with the low-carbohydrate diet makes them feel weak, depressed and irritable, hardly the best condition to be in so close to a competition. More experienced athletes have found that cutting the low-carbohydrate phase to just a single day, or skipping it completely, can be just as effective. It now appears that they may be right!

A recent study measured the muscle glycogen levels in well-trained runners after they had completed three different types of race preparation:

● The traditional carbohydrate-loading regimen of three days low-carbohydrate diet (about 100 g/4 oz of carbohydrate per day) then three days high-carbohydrate diet (550 g/19 oz of carbohydrate per day).

- Three days of normal diet (350 g/12 oz of carbohydrate per day) then three days of high-carbohydrate diet (as above).
- Three days of normal carbohydrate intake.

All the runners tapered their training over the six-day period from 90 minutes on Day 1 to complete rest on Day 6. On Day 7, before and after a performance test, muscle samples were taken to measure glycogen levels.

Simply reducing mileage, while consuming a normal diet, resulted in slightly higher than normal muscle glycogen levels. This demonstrates the importance of reducing the volume of training over the final week before competition. So the minimum you should do in preparation for competition is ensure adequate rest and a good basic diet.

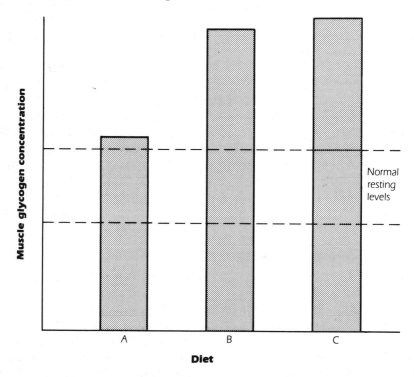

Fig.6.1 Post exercise repletion of muscle glycogen content of the quadriceps muscle following (A) a 6-day normal mixed diet (approximately 350g carbohydrate per day), (B) a mixed diet for 3 days then a high-carbohydrate diet for a further 3 days (approximately 540 g carbohydrate per day) and (C) a low-carbohydrate diet (approximately 100 g per day) for 3 days then a high-carbohydrate diet for 3 days while reducing training volume. Note that there is little difference between the (B) and (C) regimen but a pronounced difference between (A) and (B) (C).

When the carbohydrate intake was increased, considerably greater increases in muscle glycogen stores were observed. As found in earlier studies, a gradual reduction in training combined with carbohydrate restriction and then a high-carbohydrate diet resulted in muscle glycogen stores that were two to three times greater than normal. But it was particularly interesting to note that simply increasing the carbohydrate intake without having previously restricted carbohydrate intake, in combination with the training reduction (taper), resulted in comparable levels of glycogen supercompensation. In other words the degree or duration of depletion did not appear to be important in stimulating the glycogen supercompensation.

Unfortunately the exact influence of initial glycogen levels on full marathon performance remains a mystery as performance in this study was assessed only over the half-marathon distance. Although the three regimens led to differences in final muscle glycogen stores, no differences were observed in performance, which is not really surprising as it is unlikely that muscle glycogen depletion is the principal factor limiting performance in endurance activities of up to 13 miles. So, if you have ensured that your glycogen stores are normal, further increases in muscle glycogen are unlikely to be of additional benefit in competitions such as half-marathons.

What this study does tell us is that it is possible to achieve the same increases in muscle glycogen stores that are normally associated with the traditional carbohydrate-loading regimen simply by tapering your training and increasing your carbohydrate intake. And this may also be a more palatable way of increasing muscle glycogen, though it should be noted that 550–600 g/19–21 oz of carbohydrate per day is nearly twice most athletes' normal intake. So just eating a few extra biscuits or cookies and taking more sugar is not enough!

Recommendations for the taper/high-carbohydrate diet

So, should you carbohydrate-load? There is no conclusive evidence that it would improve your performance over a marathon, but it is essential in any case that you start any competition in the best possible condition; in other words, with normal or greater than normal glycogen stores. The traditional (depletion and restriction) carbohydrate-loading regimen is not a good idea for the novice competitor. Instead, a better recommendation is the taper/ high-carbohydrate diet just described. Whatever you do, try it out first — well before any important competitions.

What is the best way to take full advantage of the taper/rebound effect?

■ Ensure that your last heavy bouts of exercise are performed at least seven days before competition. Over the final week you should reduce your volume of training so that you are resting over the last two days. There is little point in attempting to cram in extra training at the last moment — you should be resting.

■ Though fasting or a high-fat diet may increase the endurance capacity of rats, there is no evidence that the same will work in humans! A poor carbohydrate intake will certainly mean low glycogen stores, so ensure that you increase your carbohydrate intake as you taper.

■ You should start increasing the amount of carbohydrate in your diet from at least five days before the event. Just because the initial studies used a three-day diet, it does not mean that three days is the optimal time-scale. It can take up to five days to achieve supercompensation, so err on the side of caution.

■ Rather than **add** foods that are high in simple, sugary carbohydrates (like confectionery, cookies and cakes) to your normal diet, which will only lead to large increases in your energy intake and body weight, you should make a fundamental switch to starchy high-carbohydrate foods. Ideally, every meal should be high in carbohydrates and this is achieved by eating foods rich in unrefined or complex carbohydrate — cereals (especially wholemeal or wholewheat bread and pasta), vegetables (particularly potatoes), fresh and dried fruit, beans and legumes. One of the additional advantages in using these foods is that you also increase your intake of vitamins, minerals and electrolytes. In any case, these foods should already be part of your normal diet and you would simply eat more of them!

■ If you overindulge in the consumption of sugary foods, you may find it difficult to maintain your appetite over the week. So save these foods for later in the week and concentrate on the starchy foods rich in complex carbohydrates. On the day before the event, you should try to eat normal quantities of food (though still high-carbohydrate, particularly late afternoon, early evening) no later because you do not want to wake up on the day of the competition feeling bloated. You may find that your weight will increase slightly but if this is the result of eating high-carbohydrate foods rather than of simple self-indulgence, this should be to your advantage, unless of course you are competing in specific weight categories (see page 115).

Avoiding diarrhoea

Stomach troubles, such as diarrhoea, are commonplace during competition, particularly abroad. Apart from being unable to eat, you will also become rapidly dehydrated, losing both water and important electrolytes from the body. It is unwise to compete in this condition as you will not be able to perform at your best and you may seriously endanger your health, so take the advice of your doctor or coach. You must try to re-establish normal body fluids and get some energy into the body. Sip plenty of fluids continuously throughout the day, ideally a dilute glucose/electrolyte solution.

Better still, don't get diarrhoea in the first place! When abroad, take care with the type of foods that you eat prior to competition. Those obviously associated with diarrhoea are shellfish and undercooked or spicy foods. It is also advisable to peel fruit and select only those foods that you are familiar with. Try to eat only in those places where the standard of hygiene is acceptable and avoid snacks from roadside vendors. When travelling abroad, why not pack some granola, muesli bars or confectionery as snacks?

No last minute training!

Do resist the temptation wherever possible for any last minute training sessions, other than the usual warm-up. Any exercise will result in some degree of glycogen utilization and may mean starting the competition with lower than normal glycogen stores.

This problem has been demonstrated in a study which measured the glycogen content of the quadriceps (thigh) muscle of a group of soccer players before, at half-time, and on completion of a game. The players naturally divided into two distinct groups (see Figure 6.2). Group A started with normal glycogen stores which were sufficient to last the duration of the match, but Group B started with lower than normal stores which were more or less depleted by half-time, meaning that they played the second half with relatively little glycogen in the working muscle. Analysis of the match clearly showed that these players covered far less distance and sprinted less than the other players — they were clearly more fatigued and their performance suffered accordingly. The had not recovered sufficiently from the previous training session to start the game in optimal condition.

Recommendations: preparing for competition

■ Do not try anything new over the week prior to competing. Rehearse your preparation routine during training sessions and at minor events. Find out what works for you.

■ Evidence does not suggest that greatly raised glycogen stores will improve performance in every sport, but it does appear that low glycogen stores are **always** a disadvantage. Make sure you start

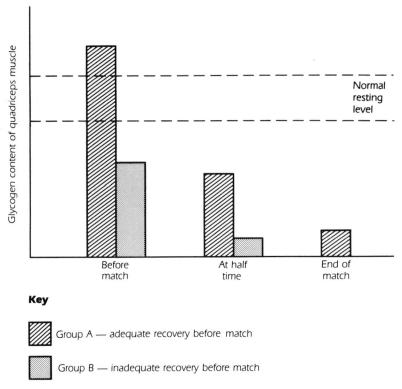

Key

Group A — adequate recovery before match

Group B — inadequate recovery before match

Fig.6.2 How adequate replenishment of muscle glycogen will influence muscle glycogen stores at the end of a game of soccer.

your competition as well prepared as possible, which means at least normal glycogen stores. This can be achieved by **both** tapering your training (reducing the rate. at which you use glycogen) **and** raising your carbohydrate intake (increasing refuelling).

■ Over the final week before competition, gradually taper your training programme and eat your normal diet (which should contain high-carbohydrate foods). Avoid any last-minute training sessions.

■ Avoid gorging at mealtimes — take smaller, more frequent high-carbohydrate meals as they are easier on the stomach.

■ Increase your fluid intake over the week to ensure you are fully hydrated **prior** to competition.

■ Avoid alcohol and unusual foods over the period leading up to competition. Save the celebrations until afterwards!

Competition day

On the day of competition, the most important thing to remember is: never try anything new. Follow a simple, sound nutritional routine: if you are competing in the morning, just eat a light carbohydrate-rich breakfast with plenty of fluids: cereal with milk, toast and jam, peanut butter or honey, or baked beans on toast are all ideal pre-event meals. Do not take large quantities of sugar, confectionery or honey — the complex carbohydrates are best. Avoid those foods you know will upset your stomach.

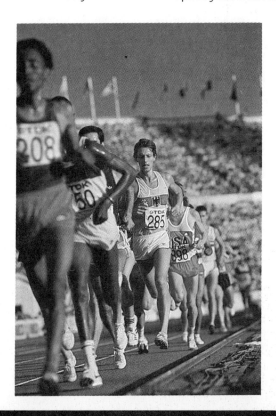

■ You should always eat something on the morning of competition as the liver glycogen stores will be depleted, even in a well-nourished, glycogen-laden individual. Anyone attempting to perform prolonged exercise with low liver glycogen stores will be less able to maintain a constant supply of glucose and so will be at a distinct disadvantage.

■ The best time to eat before competition varies between individuals: 2–3 hours would be a good general rule. You should always allow yourself several hours to digest your food fully before competing, even if this means rising slightly earlier than usual. If the event is later in the day, eat normally until 3–4 hours prior to competition and then eat a light carbohydrate-rich meal.

■ Once you have eaten, try to relax — don't rush around as this will slow down digestion. And don't eat any last minute snacks. Remember, anxiety will tend to slow the rate at which food moves out of the stomach so, while allowing 2–3 hours may have been adequate in minor events, the stress of a major competition may retard emptying. Always err on the side of caution.

■ If you cannot tolerate food, try using some of the commercial liquid meals designed specifically for sport, clinical use or simply as a meal replacement in slimming programmes, or else carbohydrate drinks in place of a meal. However, while drinks may be a useful alternative or addition to the pre-event meal, they should not be taken just prior as the principal aim is to start competing with normal blood glucose concentrations (see page 134).

■ If competing throughout the day in bouts or heats, try to take in fluids and some carbohydrate between bouts of competition. The fluid will help prevent dehydration and the carbohydrate will aid in maintaining your glycogen levels throughout the day. Once again, the emphasis should be on starchy carbohydrates rather than simple sugars, in small amounts and taken with plenty of fluid. Sandwiches with a low-fat filling (such as small amounts of honey or jam), bananas, granola or muesli bars are a good idea or alternatively try some of the commercial carbohydrate drinks specifically formulated for this purpose.

■ If competing over several days, increasing your glycogen stores prior to the first day may help to keep you going. But refuelling between competitions is vital and this can only be achieved by eating plenty of carbohydrate, preferably starchy carbohydrate. Don't wait until several hours after competition before eating — start the refuelling process immediately. And don't rely on the organizers of the event to provide the necessary foods: take responsibility and pack your own food.

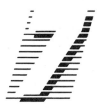

Losing and gaining weight

Principles of weight reduction

Energy balance

This concept has already been discussed in the context of muscle glycogen stores and fatigue but an understanding of 'energy balance' is also vital in appreciating the way in which diet and exercise can influence body weight and composition. Expressed in its simplest form, an individual is in energy balance when the amount of energy taken up by the body equals the amount of energy expended by the body, in other words, when **energy intake = energy output**. When intake exceeds output, something must be done with the excess energy: it must either be stored as fat or wasted in some way. If intake is less than requirement, then the additional energy needed will have to be drawn from the body's fat reserves. Even a small energy imbalance can have very pronounced effects on the composition and overall weight of the body.

One way of inducing an energy deficit is to reduce your energy intake — simply to eat less. Yet there are three problems associated with restricting energy over a long period:

- While substantially reducing the amount of energy you eat, you must continue to consume sufficient protein, vitamins, minerals and other essential nutrients — in other words, the nutrient density of each food consumed must be high, yet the energy low. If you simply eat less of the same foods, you may not be consuming sufficient nutrients, particularly if the relative balance of your diet was poor to start with. For adequate intakes of many nutrients you must eat a reasonably large amount of food each day (at least 1000 kcal/4.2 MJ of the typical Western diet). Any less and you face the risk of inadequate intakes of protein, vitamins and minerals (often referred to as hyponutrition). So you cannot stay on such a low energy intake for prolonged periods.
- Many athletes find it very difficult to lose weight while maintaining a normal training programme. Either the training suffers or they cannot continue with the diet. This failure may be attributable to over-

109

restricting energy intakes, carbohydrates in particular.

● Chronic energy restriction on its own will result in losses of tissues other than fat. It will also initiate a series of responses which reduce the energy deficit by altering energy output and thus slow down the rate at which the body fat stores are reduced. Whenever you reduce the amount of energy in your normal diet, the body is forced to call upon its long term store of energy, the fat stored under the surface of the skin. But it will try to reduce the extent of this shortage of energy via a series of complex metabolic changes which reduce the amount of energy you use in everyday life — effectively saving energy. This is an important response designed to help you survive prolonged shortages of food or starvation.

On the other hand, without altering your diet, you could increase the amount of energy you use each day by taking more exercise. Yet a very large increase in the amount of exercise alone would be required to bring about any appreciable weight loss.

The most effective and obvious way to lose weight is to do both. By combining a period of controlled energy intake and a sensible programme of endurance activity, built into your normal training programme, the difference between the amount of energy you consume and use is greatest. Not only is this the simplest way of losing weight but the extent to which you must reduce your energy intake and increase your energy usage is much less when combined together than if you altered just one of the two. Better still, the weight loss can be permanent as you will soon learn how to bring your weight under control.

Energy restriction and energy output

How does energy restriction influence energy output? The primary component of energy expenditure is the energy cost of maintaining the normal metabolic processes of the body at rest – known as the basal or resting metabolic rate (BMR). It appears that most of this energy is expended in the lean tissues of the body and muscle in particular.

One of the first consequences of caloric restriction is a reduction in BMR, possibly by as much as 15–20 per cent in the first twenty-four to forty-eight hours of dieting! This immediate response is then maintained by reducing the amount of tissue that uses energy, the lean tissue of the body. Muscle in particular, is broken down, along with fat, to provide energy. So not all of the weight you lose will be fat.

Similarly, the increases in metabolic rate that are normally observed after a meal or activity tend to be reduced — effectively preventing the body from wasting energy. The small increase in metabolic rate after a meal, often referred to as the thermic effect of feeding (TEF) or dietary-induced thermogenesis, can be divided into two parts. The first component is an obligatory energy cost (that which is required for digesting, absorbing and assimilating food), while the second appears to be independent of these processes and may represent a way of effectively wasting excess energy rather than storing it as fat. While the magnitude of TEF is very small, it may play an important part in regulating body weight over prolonged periods of time. This may explain why some people can eat very large amounts of food without putting on weight (large amounts of energy are wasted — very inefficient energy storers), while others gain weight on very low energy intakes (no energy is wasted — very efficient energy storers).

In support of this, obese individuals on weight reduction programmes and those who gain weight easily have been shown to have blunted increases in metabolic rate after feeding. Furthermore, reduced intakes of energy are often associated with a continual feeling of lethargy, tiredness and muscle weakness, which would certainly discourage you from taking any exercise and using up any more energy.

The problem with dieting

One of the problems with dieting is that you don't lose fat alone when you restrict your energy intake; you also lose water, glycogen and lean tissue. If the amount of lean tissue is a primary determinant of your basal or resting metabolic rate (BMR), then every time you lose weight by excessive dieting your BMR will also decrease, thus reducing your energy requirements still further. The BMR falls more rapidly with each successive episode of caloric restriction and the return to baseline levels takes longer each time the diet ends.

The consequence of this slowing of metabolic rate is clear. Weight reduction by dieting causes adaptive changes in energy expenditure which act to prevent further weight reduction. All these responses make it increasingly difficult to lose weight as you continue to restrict your intake of energy. Even worse, every time you fail to stick to a new weight after dieting and regain all those pounds, it will be even harder to lose weight next time as your body gets better and better at conserving energy.

Increase your total energy usage

While a single bout of exercise on its own will not use vast amounts of energy, **regular** periods of activity can be very important in increasing your total energy usage over the year. For example, even running a marathon only consumes the same amount of energy that most people eat each day (around 2500–3000 kcal/10.4–12.5 MJ). Yet, using as little as an extra 500–1000 kcal/2–4.2 MJ over the week (just 5–10 per cent of total energy intake) can add up to the equivalent of 2–9 kg/5–20 lbs of fat over the year!

Better still, regular activity will counteract those adaptations intended to save energy. Muscle will use energy in order to perform exercise and in doing so will be less likely to be used as a source of energy itself. So your metabolic rate will be less likely to fall and more of the weight that is lost will be fat, not muscle. After each bout of activity, your metabolic rate will remain elevated for some period of time. It was originally believed that the metabolic rate may go up by as much as 25 per cent for ten to fifteen hours after exercise, but recent studies suggest that the increases are more modest, around 5 per cent for two to four hours after exercise. Yet, with regular activity throughout the day and periods of exercise over the week, the general level of metabolic rate maintained will tend to be greater as it is constantly pepped up with repeated bouts of activity. This means that, even at rest, the amount of energy you use is increased. Such increases are very small but, when viewed in the long term, they all count in losing and maintaining weight.

As you lose weight and get fitter, you'll find that you can take more exercise and so be able to use more energy every time. This will help you lose weight if you continue to reduce your intake of energy or, alternatively, allow you to eat more food and yet still maintain the same weight. You'll also find that you can cope more easily with the physical challenges of training, competition and even everyday life — so improving your sense of well-being and your quality of life.

What's the best type of exercise for weight control?

The best type of exercise for weight control is any form of physical activity that you can maintain comfortably for 20–30 minutes at least three times each week. Ideally, it should be something you enjoy not endure and which naturally complements your current training programme.

There are two primary objectives to the exercise programme: to use as much energy as possible and to improve your stamina or endurance so as to benefit your cardiovascular system as much as possible. So the best form of exercise would be of low to moderate intensity with the emphasis on duration as opposed to intensity.

Remember that the number of calories you burn up depends both on how vigorous the exercise is and how long you keep it up. For example, an hour's walking uses about the same number of calories as 20 minutes' hard swimming. So, rather than rush to increase the intensity of effort as you improve, go for total time, or exercise more frequently throughout the week, and increase the intensity only when time is restricted.

Diet and training

The aim of all weight reduction diets is to restrict the food intake so that the body's fat stores are gradually reduced, while maintaining the normal body functions. This is particularly important if you want to continue training at the same level or step it up. With severe dieting, however, the weight lost over the initial few weeks is more likely to be the body's carbohydrate reserves and fluid rather than fat. Without these you will find training extremely difficult and tiring.

Most traditional weight reduction programmes advocate excluding sweet foods (such as cakes and confectionery), potatoes and bread. Although this would reduce energy intake, there would also be a drastic reduction in carbohydrate intake, so your ability to maintain muscle glycogen levels would be severely impaired, as would your capacity to exercise.

The best approach is certainly to reduce energy intake but make sure that the nutrient density, and in particular carbohydrate intake, is kept high. All your foods should be low in energy but high in carbohydrate, vitamins, minerals and trace elements (not just high in fibre). This means a high-carbohydrate, low-fat diet.

Basic changes in your diet

What sort of changes should you make? Well, if you drink, start off by cutting out alcohol altogether. It is pointless improving your eating habits if you can pour all the calories back drinking alcohol. Weight for weight, alcohol contains nearly twice as many calories as carbohydrate or protein, and watch out for the potato chips and peanuts. Try low-alcohol beers or lagers or soft drinks but not the low-carbohydrate beers as by fermenting out the sugar the alcohol content is increased. If you must take alcohol, try extending the drink with soda, lemonade or water to make it last longer. The next basic steps are to remove all visible fat from the diet (butter, oils, lard, fat on meat), substitute low-fat foods for high-fat foods (see page 11) and eat more starchy carbohydrates. If you already have a relatively low-fat diet, then you must reduce the overall quantity of food that you are consuming.

113

Don't over-restrict your energy intake

Be particularly careful of over-restricting energy intake. It is very easy to reduce gradually the amount of food eaten over long periods of weight reduction or repeated bouts of weight loss without fully appreciating just how little is eaten. The body can be conditioned into surviving on very low energy intakes, but both health and performance will suffer ultimately. The threat of hyponutrition (and possibly even disturbed eating habits requiring clinical treatment, such as anorexia) is especially evident in young female athletes who are trying to maintain low body weights (distance runners, gymnasts, etc — see Chapter 10).

Body weight

A general guide to whether you are consuming sufficient energy to match your energy expenditure is to measure your body weight. This should be measured under the same conditions on each occasion: with as little clothing as possible (preferably nude), at the same time of day (preferably on rising) and after voiding bladder and bowel. Remember that small changes in body weight (1–2 kg/2–4 lb, more in females) occur naturally — it is the general trend that is important (whether increasing, decreasing or relatively stable). Do not become fanatical about small changes on a day to day basis!

Changes in the amount of fat and muscle can occur over periods of time while the overall body weight remains constant, so a more precise means of determining body composition is required. The measurement of skinfold thicknesses (using skinfold calipers) at four sites of the body can be used to monitor changes in the thickness of the subcutaneous fat layer. As various studies have demonstrated a relationship between skinfold thickness and body density, it is possible to use these measurements to predict the amount of fat present in the body as a whole.

Not a 'diet' but a way of life

Once you have achieved your desired weight you should stick with your improved eating habits. Gradually increase the quantity of food eaten to prevent further weight loss and find out just how much food you need to maintain both your body weight and training programme. You can also **occasionally** reintroduce some of your favourite foods (such as those which contain large amounts of fat or alcohol). If your weight starts to increase again, simply revert to the weight loss regimen until it is under control.

Ideally, a longterm weight reduction programme should not be a 'diet'

114

but simply an adjustment of your relatively balanced eating habits so that you eat less. Otherwise you may eat different foods while on the 'diet' and then revert to the foods that originally made you overweight. Set yourself a realistic time frame: you should be aiming to lose around 1 kg/2 lb per week. Any more and you are not eating enough and no longer losing just fat; any less and your energy intake is still too high. This sort of weight loss can be achieved by simply reducing your energy intake by around 2100 kJ/500 kcal — not everybody should automatically go on a 4.2 MJ/1000 kcal a day diet. If you normally eat a diet providing around 12.5 MJ/3000 kcal per day and switch to around 4.2 MJ/1000 kcal, the energy deficit may be too great and both you and your training will certainly suffer. If you find you cannot maintain your training volume, you are probably over-restricting energy intake, consuming insufficient high-carbohydrate foods or simply training too hard (or all three!).

Above all, do not become paranoid about your weight loss or lack of it. Be honest with yourself, give yourself time — the best weight loss may be slow but it should also be permanent. Above all, set yourself a realistic target; there is little point in being very thin if it makes life unbearable for you and the people around you! If you can combine improvements in your eating habits with your regular training programme, you should find it comparatively easy to achieve sensible weight loss.

Finally, it should be noted that it is not possible to state 'ideal' or 'optimal' body compositions or weights for each of the various sports. While such figures are often quoted, they have been derived empirically, that is, merely on the basis of observing the body composition and weights of elite performers — little specific research has been done. These may be useful as general guidelines but they should not be applied too rigidly as most athletes are not directly comparable to elite mature performers, either in general physique or ability. They should never be applied to or enforced on young and growing children or adolescents.

Making weight

Competitors participating in sports where weight must be restricted to specified limits (combat sports, lightweight rowing, horse racing, etc) must take particular care when attempting to make weight. Many of the traditionally accepted ways of making weight, such as acute fasting, sweating out, saunas and the use of diuretics, all result in losses of glycogen and water, not fat. These regimens will always result in such large decreases in body fluids and glycogen, that it is **impossible** to rehydrate and refuel adequately prior to competition — this may take several days rather than hours! Your performance will always be impaired and, despite making

115

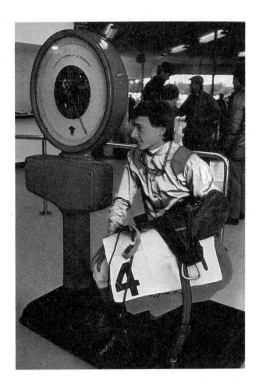

weight, you simply give your opponent a distinct advantage. A small weight advantage over your opponent, who may also have taken similar steps, is rarely worth having. Success may be determined by whose performance has suffered the least by making weight — not by who is the better competitor!

Don't make weight at the cost of performance!

The detrimental effects of such acute weight reduction programmes have been demonstrated in an American study. The consequences of the normal weight reduction programme of a group of Olympic wrestlers was observed by determining changes in muscle glycogen stores and in performance (see Table 7.1). The four-day weight reduction period (two days at 50 per cent of normal intake, followed by two days at 25 per cent food intake, plus no fluids over the final twenty-four hours) resulted in substantial decreases in muscle glycogen and muscle strength. These could not be recovered in the three hour period between weighing in and competition despite consumption of high-carbohydrate foods and large volumes of fluid. The wrestlers

	Body Weight	Muscle Glycogen	Knee Extension peak torque (Nm)		
			slow	medium	fast
	(kg)	(mmol/kg dm-^{1})			
Before	73.9	271	195	145	115
At weigh in (96H)	68.9	147	170	135	100
At competition (+3H)	71.4	168	165	135	105

Table 7.1 Influence of acute weight reduction (by restricting food and fluids) on body weight, muscle glycogen content and isokinetic strength (measured as knee extension peak torque). Source: Houston et al, 1981

had made the weight successfully and gained an apparent advantage, yet their performance was impaired!

If you have used fasting and dehydration to make the weight, then you must attempt to make up some of the deficits in water, electrolytes and carbohydrate. You may well be severely dehydrated, with low blood glucose levels (through low-liver-glycogen levels) and the amount of glycogen in your muscles will be minimal. You will probably be tired, nauseous, dizzy — hardly the best condition in which to compete. You should sip fluids containing water, electrolytes and glucose (dilute solutions only) continuously prior to competition.

The maximum weight loss that can be achieved in a relatively lean person without affecting fluid and glycogen stores is around 1 kg/2 lb per week — the rest is water and glycogen. So you should ideally be at your competition weight, or very close, at least two to three days prior to competition, preferably three to five days.

If possible, any major changes should be achieved out of the competitive season. Avoid having to lose large amounts of weight rapidly and try to train relatively close (1–2 kg/2–4 lb) to competition weight. You should not compete in a class that is well below your 'natural' weight. If you always have to lose 5 kg/11 lb or more to make weight, then you should reconsider your weight class.

One final note on making weight. The use of diuretics should be avoided at all costs. Not only will they impair your performance but they may also endanger your health.

Gaining weight

Weight can be gained by increasing either the amount of fat or the amount of muscle within your body. While increases in body fat are comparatively easy to achieve, gains in muscle mass are only attained as a result of the adaptation to intensive training. The adaptive responses to resistance training result in an anabolic state in muscles that are hypertrophying (that is, gaining in size because of an increase in function); the deposition of muscle is the result of increased protein synthesis. Because of these changes in protein metabolism, there is an increased requirement for protein. In order to assess the protein requirement of an individual it is essential that complete collections of every nitrogen-containing material from the body be made, including urine, faeces, hair, sweat, phlegm, menses and semen, and balanced against direct measurement of protein intake. But owing to the difficulties involved, very few well-controlled studies of protein requirements have ever been conducted in individuals engaging in intensive weight gain programmes. On the basis of available evidence, it is usually recommended that 1.0–1.5 g of protein per kg body weight is more than adequate to meet any increased requirement through muscle hypertrophy. As a rule, the normal dietary intake of protein (for most individuals, including the moderately active, 0.8–1.0 g of protein per kg body weight will maintain protein balance) is adequate for athletes as long as the energy intake is sufficient to maintain body weight. For example, a 70 kg/154 lb male consuming around 12.5 MJ/3000 kcal each day of a normal diet where 10–15 per cent of the energy came from protein, would consume about 75–120 g of protein per day — around 1.0–1.7 g per kg body weight.

High protein intakes will not increase muscle

Eating a high-protein diet or supplementing the diet with additional amino acids will not in itself result in any great increases in muscle mass. There is little scientific evidence that the consumption of large amounts of protein supplements will have any beneficial effects on muscle hypertrophy, muscular strength or physical performance, quite irrespective of the claims of the manufacturers (see Chapter 9). Any protein consumed in excess of requirements will simply be used as an energy source, stored as fat or excreted from the body. Every unit of protein you eat beyond your requirement is superfluous and, above all, a waste of money.

118

The common practice of eating large amounts of meat, dairy produce and eggs to increase muscle mass can be expensive. Also, it could possibly be detrimental to both your health and your performance, for two reasons:

- You are establishing abnormal eating habits which will be difficult to alter in later life and may increase the risk of coronary heart disease (see page 18).
- Eating high-protein foods leaves little appetite for the important high-carbohydrate foods. Without adequate energy intake and glycogen reserves, you will not be able to train to your full potential, and the adaptation (in this case muscle gain) will be minimal.

The best approach is to make sure that you eat a high-carbohydrate diet, so your glycogen stores are full prior to each training session. By meeting the demands of the increasing volume and quality of training, you should gain muscle mass. But if you fail to refuel adequately between sessions, you will not be able to maintain your training schedule. This is often associated with constant tiredness and with ketosis (see page 43), a sure sign that your body is not receiving sufficient carbohydrate.

Do not worry whether you are receiving sufficient amounts of essential amino acids from a normal high-carbohydrate diet. By including starchy carbohydrates in the form of grain products, legumes and nuts, along with dairy products your overall intake of essential amino acids with carbohydrate, vitamins and minerals will remain adequate.

While you should ideally try to limit your weight gain so that only muscle mass is increased, this is rarely achieved in practice. It is probably easier to accept the small increases in fat stores associated with weight gain and then reduce them once the desired muscle mass has been attained. But be careful that you don't simply overeat!

Summary

- An individual is in energy balance when energy intake equals energy output.

- The most effective way to lose weight is to combine a period of controlled energy intake and a sensible programme of endurance activity into your normal training programme.

- The aim of all weight reduction diets is to restrict food intake so that the body's fat stores are gradually reduced, while maintaining the normal body functions. However, nutrient density (of nutrients other than fat) in particular carbohydrate intake, should be kept high.

- Fat and alcohol contain nearly twice as many calories as carbohydrate or protein, so alcohol and foods high in fat should be deleted from a weight-reducing diet.

- It is important not to over-restrict your energy intake on a weight-reducing diet as this will impair performance and health.

- You should be aiming to lose around 1 kg/2 lb per week on a weight-reducing diet. Any more and you are no longer losing just fat. Any less and your energy intake is too high.

- Don't make weight at the cost of performance.

- Weight can be gained by increasing either the amount of fat or the amount of muscle within your body.

- As a rule, the normal dietary intake of protein is adequate for athletes, as long as the energy intake is sufficient to maintain body weight. Eating a high protein diet or supplementing the diet with additional amino acids will not result in any great increases in muscle mass.

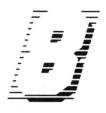

Vitamins and minerals

Vitamins

Vitamins are substances that the body needs in very small amounts, but cannot make for itself in sufficient quantities, if at all. They are complex organic substances that act principally as regulators of a wide variety of processes essential for normal metabolism, growth and the development of the human body.

Those vitamins involved in energy metabolism are rather like the spark plugs of an engine. They do not contain energy in themselves but they play essential roles in metabolic reactions which are responsible for harnessing, storing and using energy in the body (see Figure 8.1).

The discovery of the 'vital amine'

In the 1890s, a Dutch scientist studying a disease called **beriberi** in Indonesia found that he could induce the disease in chickens simply by restricting their diet to polished rice which was the staple food in areas where the disease was endemic. If he added the husks of the rice (removed during polishing) back to the diet, the disease was cured. There was clearly some vital factor essential for life present in the husk but omitted from the polished rice.

A Polish biochemist suggested that there was just one vital factor, a chemical called an amine, hence his term, 'vital amine' or 'vitamine'. Even when a whole variety of other factors were discovered, the term (with the final 'e' dropped) was applied to them all.

From then on, the discovery of new vitamins became a scientific craze with the discovery of over fifty during the first half of this century. Some were correctly identified, most wrongly — resulting in terminological confusion. The original 'vitamine' was shown to be two vitamins: one was soluble in organic solvents, the other soluble in water. These were termed A and B. Vitamins C and D soon joined the collection, while B was found to consist of several different kinds named, naturally, B_1, B_2 and up to B_{20}. The same thing happened in other groups.

Of the original fifty or more substances first thought to be essential in the

Vitamin		Good sources	Involved in
A	Retinol or carotene	Liver, dairy produce, eggs, carrots, green leafy veg	Visual processes, connective tissue, skin
B₁	Thiamin	Meat, whole grains, legumes, nuts	Carbohydrate metabolism, CNS function
B₂	Riboflavin	Liver, dairy produce, meat, cereal	Carbohydrate metabolism, vision, skin
B₆	Pyridoxin	Meat, fish, green leafy veg, whole grains, legumes	Protein metabolism, red blood cell formation, CNS function
B₁₂	Cyano-cobalamin	Meat, fish, dairy produce; No vegetable sources	Red blood cell formation, CNS function
—	Niacin	Liver, meat, fish, peanuts, cereal products	Carbohydrate and fat metabolism
—	Folic acid	Liver, legumes, green leafy veg	Regulates growth of cells, including red blood cells
C	Ascorbic acid	Green leafy veg, fruit, potatoes, white bread	Connective tissue, iron absorption/metabolism, healing/infection
D	Calciferols	Dairy produce, action of sunlight on skin	Calcium metabolism, bones and teeth
E	Tocopherols	Vegetable oils, liver, green leafy veg, dairy produce, whole grains	Protects vitamins A & C, and fatty acids, from destruction in body (anti-oxidant)
K	—	Green leafy veg and liver	Clotting of blood, fat digestion

Table 8.1 The principal sources and functions of vitamins.

diet, the list has now been reduced to just twelve, although there are some others which may also be important as they are essential to life in other species (for example, choline, inositol, bioflavonoids and carnitine). Of the

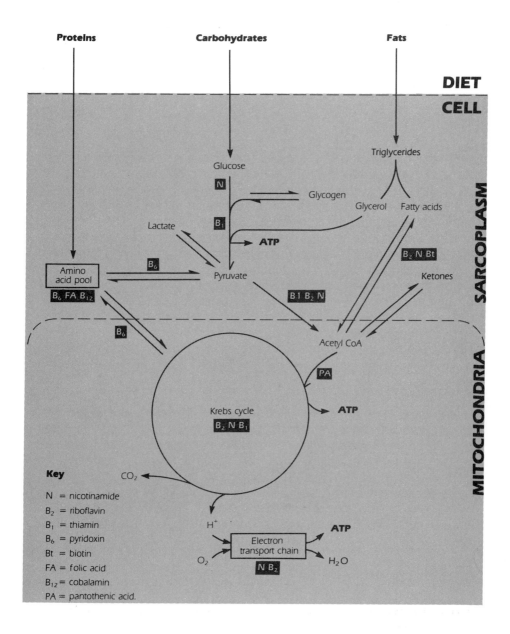

Fig.8.1 The importance of vitamins in cellular metabolism. Superimposed on Figure 2.7, it is quite clear that vitamins have a vital role to play in nutrient metabolism.

series of B vitamins, only B_1, B_2, B_6 and B_{12} were found to be separate vitamins. As their chemical composition became better understood, names were ascribed (such as pyridoxine for B_6 and cyanocobalamin for B_{12}) and sometimes the compounds were found to be metabolically and functionally related (the group of compounds called tocopherols or Vit E, for example).

Vitamin storage

The fat-soluble vitamins (A,D,E and K) are stored in large amounts in body tissues (particularly the liver). So extensive are the stores that it may take several months or even years before a fat-soluble vitamin deficiency arises in a previously well-nourished individual. Excessive intakes of these vitamins continue to accumulate, saturating all body stores and resulting in cellular damage. Excessive amounts of A, for example, can cause liver damage, while overdosing with D can increase the body's absorption and handling of calcium, leading to cellular damage in the kidney, liver and heart.

In contrast, the water-soluble vitamins are not stored well in the body and any intake in excess of requirements is generally excreted in the urine. This relatively small store of water-soluble vitamins also explains why deficiency states can arise rapidly (in as little as one or two months). While these vitamins tend to be non-toxic when taken in moderate excess, very large amounts of certain vitamins have been found to interact with the absorption and utilization of other nutrients (C, for example), impair liver function (nicotinic acid) and nerve function (B_6).

Illness as a result of vitamin deficiency is comparatively rare in the West nowadays. Just by eating a **variety** of different foods, it is possible to get an adequate supply of most vitamins — it is not necessary to eat vast quantities of green vegetables or liver. The way in which food is stored and prepared, however, can reduce its vitamin content, but as long as the emphasis is placed upon fresh produce which is cooked quickly (without being kept warm for long periods or reheated), the vitamin levels in a normal diet are still very much above our daily requirements.

Vitamin supplementation and performance

There is little evidence to indicate that, in general, the diets of athletes are specifically low in any particular vitamin or that athletes show clinical or biochemical signs of vitamin deficiency. Yet recent surveys have shown that 30–80 per cent of athletes regularly take vitamin and mineral supplements of one form or another throughout training and competition. In using such supplements, many believe that performance will be enhanced. This is often based on the assumption that, as certain vitamins are involved in energy metabolism, consumption of more of a particular vitamin will improve performance by providing extra energy. Is there any evidence that supplementing the diet with specific vitamins will improve athletic perform- ance? A vast number of studies have been conducted on this aspect of sports nutrition but, when reviewing the available literature, the most consistent finding is that supplementation has no significant effect on performance. Also, as it is accepted that vitamin deficiency impairs performance, this lack of effect must also be taken to indicate that the subjects in these studies were already receiving sufficient amounts of the vitamin in the diet.

Where improvements in performance have been reported, two explana- tions are possible. Either supplementation did, in fact, lead to improved performance, or the subjects were initially vitamin-deficient and supple- mentation restored performance to the level associated with normal vitamin stores. One other factor that should not be overlooked is the power of the mind — 'the placebo effect' — whereby the psychological effects of giving the supplement are observed rather than any nutritional benefits. So whether the excessive intake of vitamin supplements leads to improvements in performance remains open to debate, but appears doubtful.

Vitamin deficiency in athletes

There is little hard scientific evidence to suggest that the utilization, destruction or excretion of vitamins is increased with sporting activities, though it must be stated that there have been relatively few well-controlled studies using elite and high-level performers specifically to assess vitamin needs and the nutritional status of the athlete. There is some evidence to suggest that B requirements (especially B_2) may increase with regular intensive exercise. But the greater energy expenditure of athletes is normally associated with an increased consumption of food in general, leading to higher than normal intakes of these vitamins — especially if whole grain cereal products rich in carbohydrate are eaten. On the other hand, those who eat relatively little and train hard may be disadvantaged.

Certain factors other than your diet or your exercise regimen may also influence your requirements for certain vitamins:

- Excessive alcohol intake may impair absorption of B_1, folic acid, B_{12} and C.
- Regular large doses of aspirin and other anti-inflammatories may reduce C levels.

125

- Oral contraceptives tend to deplete the body's stores of folic acid, B_1, B_2, B_6 and C.
- Smoking increases the need for C and interferes with B_1 and B_{12} metabolism.

Unfortunately, as most athletes in intensive training can readily identify with the symptoms associated with vitamin deficiencies, such as fatigue, depression, weakness and muscular aches, many take this to mean that they have a deficiency state. These are, however, the natural consequences of physical exercise, so it is highly unlikely that taking additional vitamins, on top of a varied diet consumed in reasonable quantities, will reduce the severity of these symptoms or suddenly increase the supply and utilization of energy.

So why do athletes use supplements so willingly? The answer is probably: hope, combined with vigorous and effective commercial promotion. As with most advertising, the promotion of vitamins is carefully controlled by advertising standards regulations. Manufacturers are not permitted to suggest that vitamins will cure or prevent disease, and they must be able to provide valid evidence to support any claims they do make. In sport, unfortunately, the in-house promotion of such products in limited circulation magazines and by word of mouth through pyramid-type selling means that the claims of many products go unchallenged. Consequently, great powers are commonly attributed to certain vitamins even when scientific evidence is totally lacking. Vast profits can be made simply by relying on the ignorance and nutritional naivety of the consumer.

Increasing vitamin intakes

There may be certain instances, though, where specific attempts to increase vitamin intakes through alterations in diet or through supplementation may be warranted. The poor eating habits of some athletes may result in limited vitamin intakes and suboptimal stores of certain nutrients, as with many other young people not involved in sport.

More specifically, those participating in combat sports, lightweight rowers and jockeys competing within specific weight limits, as well as young female distance runners, gymnasts and dancers, may all be continually restricting their food intake in order to maintain low body weights (see page 81). In these circumstances it is important to consume foods of high nutrient density (particularly vitamins and iron) in order to prevent the consequences of hyponutrition.

Similarly, the female athlete who experiences a heavy menstrual flow may also have increased requirements for iron and those vitamins associated with

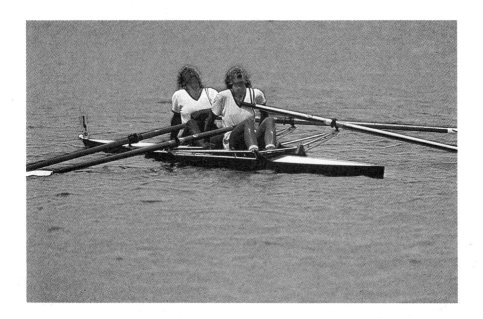

blood formation. She should seek medical assistance in monitoring her haematological (blood) status and adjust her diet or use commercial iron preparations accordingly.

It may be justified in such instances to take a single proprietary multivitamin–multimineral supplement on a daily basis. But before supplementing a poor diet with specific nutrients, efforts should first be made to improve or correct those eating habits responsible for the shortage. In most instances, any shortages of nutrients are more likely to be the result of inadequate intake rather than an increased requirement through exercise.

Vitamin overdoses

While a small extra dose of vitamins will usually do no harm, larger doses (as just mentioned) can sometimes have detrimental effects on health and can even be fatal! Most foods that we eat contain vitamins in relatively small amounts and, while there are certain items that are very high in specific vitamins (for example, cod liver oil, red palm oil, and polar bear liver are all extremely rich sources of the fat-soluble vitamins) we eat such foods rarely, if at all! So by eating **food**, it is relatively difficult to overdose on vitamins. On the other hand, thanks to technology, man is now capable of either concentrating or synthesizing vitamins in such quantities that it is very easy to consume intakes in tablet form that are 10–1000 times what could be consumed in food. The use of megavitamin preparations means that the body can be exposed to non-physiological doses of vitamins exceeding the capabilities of the body to deal with them, so leading to cellular damage and even, with some vitamins, death.

You should note that so-called 'natural' vitamins are generally no better than synthetic ones: the chemical structure is nearly always the same. Neither do 'organic' vitamins have any special properties. There is little evidence that time-released or specially coated types of vitamin are any more efficient or effective than the ordinary variety.

Minerals

Approximately 5 per cent of our body is composed of minerals. In addition to forming its basic structure (via calcium in our skeleton), minerals are also essential to the maintenance of nerve and muscle function and many serve as catalysts helping enzymes to do their work, so they are vital for normal metabolism. Consequently, abnormal mineral metabolism can have dramatic and severe physiological results.

Minerals fall broadly into two groups:

● Macrominerals are those needed in relatively large amounts (around 100 mg per day), and including calcium, magnesium, sodium, potassium and chloride.
● Trace elements are required in much smaller daily amounts (less than 2–5 mg) and include iron, copper, zinc, manganese, iodine, sulphur, cobalt, chromium and selenium. Although required in small amounts, these trace elements often interact with the macrominerals.

It is becoming increasingly apparent that our understanding of the role and metabolism of minerals, and trace elements in particular, is incomplete, and more research is required. In the light of these gaps in our knowledge, the best advice is to ensure that your intake of these nutrients is adequate by eating a varied diet rich in unrefined foods.

Of the minerals, the most important in relation to the athlete is likely to be iron.

Iron

Although technically a trace element, iron is generally considered to be a major nutrient because of its important role in metabolism. Despite the fact

Mineral	Sources	Involved in
Sodium	Salt, cheese, muscle/organ meat, fish/bacon	Neuromuscular transmission (nerve conduction) fluid and acid-base balance
Potassium	Meat, milk, veg, cereals, nuts	Neuromuscular transmission (nerve conduction) fluid and acid-base balance
Calcium	Milk, cheese, nuts, green veg, bread	Bone/tooth structure Nerve conduction, blood clotting
Magnesium	Green veg, meats, dairy produce, cereals	Neuromuscular transmission Bone formation, enzyme reactions – energy metabolism
Phosphorus	Grains and cereals, meat, milk, green veg	Bone/tooth formation, energy metabolism
Iron	Nuts/seeds, red muscle/organ meat, eggs, green veg	Haemoglobin/myoglobin formation
Zinc	Muscle meats, seafood, green veg	Enzyme synthesis
Copper	Shellfish, organ meats, nuts legumes, cocoa/chocolate	Enzyme synthesis
Iodine	Seafood, eggs, dairy produce	Thyroid function
Fluoride	Seafood, water, tea	Tooth structure
Manganese	Nuts, dried fruit, cereals/grains, tea	Enzyme synthesis
Chromium	Meat and dairy products, eggs	Glucose/insulin metabolism
Selenium	Seafood, organ and muscle meats and grains	Anti-oxidant (membranes) electron transfer

Table 8.2 The principal sources and functions of minerals.

that some 5 per cent of the earth's crust is iron, iron deficiency is one of the most prevalent disorders in the Western world.

Iron is an essential constituent of the haemoglobin found in the red blood cell, myoglobin (the equivalent oxygen-carrying compound in muscle) and many of the enzymes involved in the energy-yielding pathways in the mitochondria. So it plays a vital role in maintaining the oxygen transport system and the capacity to perform muscular work.

Iron deficiency anaemia can therefore cause marked impairments in physical performance, particularly in endurance activities. Anaemia with low haemoglobin levels would clearly impair oxygen transport yet it is also possible to be iron-deficient without being anaemic and there have been many reports of athletes exhibiting signs of inadequate iron intake.

Whether iron deficiency without anaemia will result in impairments in performance is uncertain. But as iron deficiency often predisposes an individual to anaemia, it should be avoided. Many studies have identified endurance runners, both males and females, and sportswomen in general (see Chapter 10) as particularly at risk: many have depleted iron stores without overt clinical signs of anaemia. Inadequate iron intake results in loss of strength and endurance, easy fatigability, shortened attention span and loss of visual perception — all vital attributes for sport.

A number of factors may contribute to the iron deficiency and lowered haemoglobin levels often reported in athletes, a phenomonen often referred to as 'sports anaemia':

- Increased iron losses may be associated with heavy sweating, heavy menstrual blood flow or decreased absorption from the gut.
- There may also be increased destruction of red blood cells and excretion of haemoglobin in the urine due to mechanical trauma or a decreased rate of haemoglobin synthesis through deficiencies of protein, B_{12}, folic acid or iron.
- Athletes on low energy intakes (such as those controlling their body weights) may often consume insufficient iron in the diet.
- Low iron levels may also be a natural response to endurance training which has resulted in an increase in blood volume for the same number of red blood cells (simply a dilution effect).

The iron-deficient athlete should be identified and receive professional dietary counselling and supplementation where necessary. Better still, steps should be taken to prevent iron-deficiency from the outset, prevention always being better than cure. General dietary advice would emphasize iron-rich foods of both animal and vegetable origin. If inadequate iron is consumed despite attention to the diet, then a low-level iron supplement may be beneficial in maintaining longterm iron status. It should be noted that, if all other causes of anaemia have been eliminated and sports anaemia persists, no treatment is believed to be necessary.

While increasing iron intake would clearly benefit the iron-deficient athlete, is there any value in supplementing the diet of non-deficient athletes? There is little evidence that additional iron will increase the number of red blood cells or the oxygen-carrying capacity in a non-deficient athlete, or enhance performance in any way.

The body conserves much of its iron by recycling it (30–40 mg every day) from old blood cells to new. Losses, mainly in sweat and urine, account for around 1 mg per day (although menstrual losses would increase this figure). As we only absorb about 10 per cent of the iron we consume, we need at least 10 mg per day to replace that lost from the body. So the recommended daily amount of iron is 12–15 mg per day for females and 10 mg for males. To achieve this amount, the diet must provide at least 8–10 mg of iron for every 4.2 MJ/1000 kcal. But as many people eat less than 6.3 MJ/1500 kcal or include large amounts of highly processed foods which dilute the nutrients in the diet, many athletes consequently fail to consume adequate amounts of iron.

Part of the solution is to eat more foods rich in iron:

- There is no escaping the fact that one of the best sources of iron is red meats, and liver in particular — a single serving of liver provides 10–30 mg. If you don't like the idea of a large piece of liver on your dinner plate, why not slice it into thin strips and serve it in a risotto or some other rice dish.
- Unrefined foods, like whole grains and beans, are also good sources of iron.
- Unfortunately, the absorption of iron from vegetables is relatively poor compared with that from red meats or liver, but it can be improved by eating green leafy vegetables along with cereals, rice and beans as vitamin C helps increase iron absorption.

So, by making sure your caloric intake stays high, eating lots of beans, green leafy vegetables and whole grains, with the occasional serving of liver, it is possible to satisfy our requirements for iron quite comfortably.

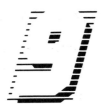

Pills, powders and potions

There is no dispute that the most effective way of enhancing athletic performance is through systematic and consistent training. Nutrition makes its greatest impact by supporting this process as, through training, comes adaptation and improvements in strength, power or endurance. Despite all this, you only need look at any sports magazine to note the vast array of nutritional products claiming to be 'specifically formulated to improve performance'. These nutritional 'ergogenic aids' (from the Greek **ergon** meaning work) theoretically permit an individual to accomplish more physical work than would otherwise be possible.

There is an enormous range of nutritional substances used as ergogenic aids in sport. Many have absolutely no proven value or even any scientific basis for their claimed effectiveness: they rely simply on folklore and consumer ignorance (green-lipped mussel extract, for example). At the other end of the spectrum, some products are based on fundamentally sound scientific principles and have in fact been shown to enhance performance in the laboratory (carbohydrate ingestion during exercise, for example).

Even at best, the improvements in performance associated with using ergogenic aids are minimal compared with those produced by training. But from the athletes' viewpoint, if they have been training continually at the upper limits of physical performance for some time, the amount of work required to achieve any further improvements in performance is considerable. So any improvements through the use of supplements would appear advantageous — hence their popularity.

The use of non-nutritional ergogenic aids (such as anabolic steroids, blood doping or hypnosis) is beyond the scope of this chapter. This discussion will therefore concentrate on those substances believed to influence performance via nutrition. These can be broadly classified as follows:

- Those substances which help replace diminishing reserves of energy during exercise, essentially providing additional carbohydrate to supplement depleted fuel stores.
- Those which can be used to assist in the recovery processes following exercise, in particular food or energy concentrates designed to enhance glycogen repletion.

- Those, such as caffeine, which alter the relative utilization of fuels during exercise.
- Those, such as alkalizing agents, which are believed to influence the accumulation of the end-products of metabolism, thereby influencing the fatigue process.
- The miscellaneous collection of extracts of herbs, minerals and animal products believed to influence performance, such as ginseng, royal jelly, etc.

Supplementing fuel stores during exercise

Dehydration and depletion of the body's reserves of carbohydrate are two of the primary limitations to maintaining high rates of energy utilization for prolonged periods. The possibility that fatigue may be offset by consuming additional carbohydrate in liquid form during exercise has consequently led to the commercial development of many sports nutrition drinks. Many companies also advertise that the drink contains the essential minerals lost in sweat that will prevent cramp, hence the development of 'electrolyte replacement drinks' containing both electrolytes and carbohydrate (normally glucose).

Electrolytes

As the primary purpose of drinking while exercising is to provide water to replace body fluids lost through sweating, any sports drink must ensure that fluid absorption during exercise is maximized and never compromised. Yet, one of the principal factors governing gastric emptying and fluid absorption is the osmolality (relative concentration) of the solution (see page 88). When we drink, the osmolality will determine the movement of fluid into the body:

- If the drink is too concentrated (or hypertonic), water will move from the body's fluid into the gut to dilute the ingested solution ie, water is secreted rather than absorbed.
- If the concentration of the drink is less concentrated than that of body fluids (or hypotonic), water molecules will move from the gut into the body.

So adding various electrolytes or glucose to water will obviously increase the osmolality of the solution. Each electrolyte will contribute two particles, while non-electrolyte substances, such as glucose, yield only one particle.
It should be noted that the presence of **very small** amounts of glucose,

133

Na$^+$ and Cl$^-$ ions in solution (eg a hypotonic solution) will actually promote the movement of water accross the gut — thus enhancing fluid intake. However, if the amounts of carbohydrate and electrolytes are greatly increased in an attempt to provide more energy or electrolytes, the absorption of water will therefore be compromised.

There appears to be little need to replace the electrolytes lost in sweat during exercise (see page 92) and, while the underlying mechanisms are not well understood, there is no evidence that cramp will either be prevented or be cured by the ingestion of electrolyte solutions or salt tablets. Adding excessive amounts of electrolytes will only elevate osmolality and retard emptying (although there is some evidence that very small amounts of Na$^+$ and Cl$^-$ ions promote fluid absorption in the intestine). So, rather than considering such drinks as replacing electrolytes, they should be viewed as fluid replenishment drinks which may also supplement the body's energy reserves.

Carbohydrate

The addition of carbohydrate to water will reduce the rate of gastric emptying since **all** sugars have a retarding effect, regardless of whether the drink contains glucose, fructose or sugar. While **very dilute** solutions are still emptied from the stomach at near maximal rates, increasing the glucose concentration to anywhere above 3–5 per cent (3–5 g per 100 ml) dramatically slows the rate of emptying. For example, 15 minutes after drinking 400 ml of plain water, 60–70 per cent of the volume would usually have emptied from the stomach. In contrast only 5 per cent of an equal volume of a 10 per cent sucrose solution (comparable to a commercial carbonated drink) would have left the stomach.

One of the limitations of using simple sugars as the carbohydrate source in these drinks is that the total amount of carbohydrate delivered to the body at such low concentrations is unlikely to make a significant contribution to energy provision during exercise. Recent studies have shown, however, that certain forms of carbohydrates may be delivered to the intestine faster than others.

Glucose polymers and maltodextrins

Since the osmolality of the drink is one of the prime factors affecting gastric emptying, a carbohydrate that has fewer particles in solution than another for the same amount of energy will empty faster. As both a single glucose molecule and a polymer of glucose molecules joined together will each contribute one particle, considerably more carbohydrate and energy can be delivered by the latter for the same osmolality. Glucose polymers (called glucose syrups and maltodextrins) are obtained from the partial digestion of corn starch and can provide as much as ten times the energy of the simple sugars for the same osmolality without slowing the rate of gastric emptying.

Recent studies have described the effect of consuming maltodextrins in sports drinks on endurance performance. Research in Texas showed that exercise time to exhaustion at a brisk walk (about 45 per cent $\dot{V}O_2max$) was increased by 11 per cent over that observed when plain water was ingested. Comparable improvements in run time to exhaustion at marathon-type pace (or slightly higher, 85 per cent $\dot{V}O_2max$) have also been reported by several independent research groups. One group from the Philippines found that, when no water was permitted, the subjects were able to run for about 56 minutes before becoming exhausted: with water they were able to run for 78 minutes. (This 40 per cent improvement demonstrates the importance of taking fluid during exercise.) When, however, the subjects drank a maltodextrin solution rather than water they were able to run for 102 minutes, an improvement of 30 per cent over that observed on water alone. It should be noted, however, that no other studies have observed such marked improvements in performance.

The potential value of drinks such as maltodextrin solutions in sporting activities (where it is the rate of work that is important rather than the ability to continue for longer) has yet to be established. However, in the absence of specific performance studies during competition, some insight into the potential benefits has been shown by another Texas study. If was found that approximately 12 per cent more work could be performed on a cycle ergometer over a two-hour period (particularly over the final 10 minutes of the trial) when the subjects drank a maltodextrin solution, in comparison to plain water. The improved performances in each study were attributed to a greater supply of energy from the carbohydrate provided in the drink.

Glucose and water intake

While the consumption of glucose may have a principal role in the supplementation of the liver's capacity to maintain blood glucose levels, it appears to have little effect on performance unless the glucose output of the liver is already inadequate to support glucose uptake by the muscle (that is, where hypoglycaemia has limited performance). This suggests that energy drinks are not as beneficial in practical terms as generally assumed unless the activity is truly prolonged (lasting more than two hours).

In fact, excessive intakes of glucose either just prior to or during exercise may severely impair performance! Taking sugared drinks, glucose tablets or confectionery in the 30–60 minutes prior to exercise leads to rapid increases in blood glucose concentration (hyperglycaemia) and the release of insulin from the pancreas. If exercise is initiated with high insulin levels, glucose is rapidly transported into the cells, resulting in a rapid fall in blood glucose beyond normal resting values (hypoglycaemia) and this promotes fatigue. Similarly, taking large amounts of glucose during exercise not only limits fluid absorption but the elevated insulin levels will inhibit fat mobilization, thus placing an even greater dependency on the limited reserves of glycogen. Both of these lead to earlier fatigue during endurance events. This inhibitory effect of glucose on fat mobilization may be countered if small amounts of glucose are given regularly throughout exercise, once the individual has been exercising for some 30–45 minutes, as the insulin response is much reduced as exercise proceeds.

Fructose is often used in sports drinks as it is believed to be transported directly to the liver and metabolized to glucose. It may be used directly by the liver for energy or released as glucose or stored as glycogen within the liver without producing a rise in plasma insulin, thus permitting fat mobilization. But only very small amounts of fructose can be tolerated in the gut without major disturbances (such as diarrhoea) so its use is limited.

The twin quests for water and glucose during exercise are therefore to some extent mutually exclusive. The greater the glucose content of the drink, the less water will be absorbed and vice versa. It appears that the delivery of carbohydrate into the intestine is relatively unaffected by the concentration of carbohydrate in solution. Dilute drinks will deliver the same amount of carbohydrate as very concentrated drinks but with considerably more water. So the practical advice is as follows:

- Satisfy the primary need — either fluids or energy.

- Choose weak diluted drinks when fluid replacement is most important, such as on hot days or when training and competing in a hot humid indoor environment.

- On cool days, during winter sports or when relatively low intensities of activity are sustained for very long periods, sweat losses are less and dehydration less of a threat. The carbohydrate content of the drink can then be increased, delivering more energy at the expense of fluids.

- Used following or between bouts of exercise (such as in a tournament), a drink providing both carbohydrate and fluid would theoretically help promote recovery. It would offset the progressive depletion of glycogen stores associated with competition throughout the day or over successive days.

Glycogen repletion

The rate at which glycogen is repleted following exercise is dependent in part upon the continual supply of dietary carbohydrate, and very large amounts of food need to be eaten to satisfy this demand (see page 81). This situation is often encountered in preparation for competition when elevated glycogen stores are desired, or during a tournament lasting several days when there is limited time available to refuel.

In such circumstances, the use of a carbohydrate concentrate, at best providing all the necessary B vitamins that would normally be associated with that amount of carbohydrate as well, may be beneficial. This would ideally supplement the ordinary high-carbohydrate diet with at least an additional 100 g/4 oz of carbohydrate. This in itself would only provide around 400 kcal/1700 kJ but would substantially increase your carbohydrate intake. The concentrate would be taken **with** a meal — rather than before or instead of — so the intake of nutrients would be unimpaired. Such supplements should not necessarily become a basic part of your diet in everyday life, but used in special circumstances:

- At times when the stresses placed on the body's limited glycogen reserves are so great that glycogen stores are still progressively depleted in spite of a diet rich in carbohydrates
- When preparing for competition

When an individual is unable to consume food for prolonged periods due to depressed appetite, such as during recovery from illness, there is a risk of general hyponutrition. Under these extreme circumstances, an easily digested liquid meal containing a balance of all nutrients — protein, carbohydrate, fats, vitamins, minerals and trace elements — may be more beneficial than just providing carbohydrates. The liquid meal does not have to be formulated specifically for sport as there are many such meal replacement products available.

Altered fuel utilization

The provision of energy during prolonged submaximal exercise is derived from a mixture of carbohydrate (as glycogen or glucose) and fat (as free fatty acids). As fatigue often appears to be related to the depletion of muscle glycogen reserves, anything enabling you to maintain the same pace while deriving a greater proportion of energy from free fatty acids would be theoretically advantageous — so effectively mimicking endurance training.

As the primary adaptation to endurance training is a shift towards fat metabolism (sparing glycogen and delaying fatigue), some studies have attempted to increase fat utilization by making more free fatty acids available during exercise. In the laboratory, numerous methods have been tried in order to raise the fatty acid concentration in blood (such as drinking corn oil and infusing the anticoagulant heparin into the circulation). While they resulted in enhanced fat oxidation, they are generally impractical or unsafe to use in sport. Consuming triglycerides during exercises has been found not only to be highly unpalatable but also to have no discernible effect on fuel utilization or performance. Similarly, ingesting glycerol as an additional gluconeogenic substrate was also found to have no impact on performance as humans do not appear to be able to convert glycerol to glucose fast enough for it to be of any practical value during exercise.

Caffeine

The perceived potential advantages of coffee ingestion on endurance performance (so often promoted by coffee manufacturers at marathons) stem from reports that caffeine increases fatty acid utilization during prolonged submaximal exercise. Caffeine affects numerous physiological systems, including skeletal muscle, the fat cells (adipocytes) and the nervous system. By increasing the release of free fatty acids from adipocytes into the circulation, more fat is oxidized.

Some studies have clearly demonstrated a corresponding glycogen-sparing effect and increased endurance time to exhaustion in the laboratory. In one study, for example, trained cyclists achieved 7 per cent more work over two hours when given caffeine compared with their performance on placebo. Another study found that cross-country skiers completed a 23 km (14 mile) course lasting about 50 minutes some 2–3 per cent faster using caffeine. Although caffeine appears to improve performance during prolonged endurance activities, it has been found to be ineffective in promoting high-intensity activities lasting less than 10 minutes. Such activities are less dependent upon fat as a fuel, so any increase in fat metabolism would be less advantageous.

Unfortunately there are disadvantages associated with caffeine ingestion:

- The amount of caffeine required to produce the reported effects is considerable, amounting to several cups of strong black coffee.
- Apart from stimulating fat mobilization, caffeine is also a powerful central nervous system stimulant and people have different thresholds of sensitivity. For some people this is so low that they cannot take caffeine in any quantity without suffering headaches, nausea, etc.

- Overdoses of caffeine reduce the perception of fatigue and affect neuromuscular efficiency, so the consumption of unusually large amounts could be detrimental to performance.
- Caffeine is a strong diuretic and anything accelerating the loss of fluids and electrolytes from the body during exercise is disadvantageous. Without sufficient body fluids, your ability to cool the body through sweating is impaired and you could overheat. Both of these effects would greatly outweigh any potential benefits of coffee ingestion as well as possibly ruining your chances of completing the competition!
- Finally, caffeine is included on the list of banned substances by the International Olympic Committee.

Therefore it would **not** be advisable for anybody to use large amounts of caffeine for the first time prior to competition — even taken as coffee. If you want to use caffeine, try it out in training and make sure it works for you, but be careful. One final point: most people take milk and sugar in their coffee. The insulin response to increases in blood glucose would swamp the caffeine effect, thereby negating any potential benefits!

End-product accumulation

One of the primary causes of fatigue during brief high-intensity exercise lasting less than 5–10 minutes is believed to be the accumulation of hydrogen ions generated by the incomplete combustion of glycogen in muscle (see page 40). The rate at which hydrogen ions accumulate in muscle is dependent on their rate of production and rate of removal from the muscle. As the concentration of hydrogen ions increases, acidity rises markedly and the capacity of the muscle to perform exercise is impaired.

There are two main ways of clearing hydrogen ions from muscle:

- 'Mopping up' the hydrogen ions by using buffers within the muscle. This capacity appears to be increased by interval training so that more work can be performed before the detrimental consequences of increased muscle acidity are experienced.
- The hydrogen ions may leave the muscle to enter the circulation where they can be 'mopped up' by the blood's own buffering systems. The movement of hydrogen ions out of the muscle depends in part on the acidity of the blood which is in turn dependent on how well the blood's buffering system has removed hydrogen ions.

Animal studies have shown that making the blood more alkaline increases the rate at which hydrogen ions leave the muscle, lowers the rate of hydrogen ion accumulation in the muscle and so reduces fatigue. Consuming sodium bicarbonate solutions in an attempt to reproduce this effect in humans — and thereby improve athletic performance — have proved inconclusive. No improvements in performance have been observed during all-out bursts of maximal effort lasting less than 60 seconds despite altering the initial acidity of the blood. However, some improvements in performance — in duration of work rather than rate of work — have been seen during activities at lower exercise intensities lasting 5–15 minutes, and during repeated bouts of high-intensity exercise. This suggests that oral alkalizing agents only influence performance in activities where there is sufficient time and blood flow to remove hydrogen ions from the working muscle. When the exercise intensity is great and the duration short, as in sprinting, the rate at which hydrogen ions accumulate and fatigue occurs is too great to be altered by changes in hydrogen ion outflow.

So it would appear that oral alkalizing agents, such as sodium bicarbonate solutions, may enhance performance in certain activities — particularly intermittent sprints or bursts of energy over periods of 2–15 minutes. However, the improvements are relatively small and the use of such substances should be established initially in training rather than in competition.

Miscellaneous substances

Over the years, a wide variety of different foods or compounds have been proposed as ergogenic aids. These include honey, royal jelly, bee pollen, lecithin, gelatin, wheat germ oil and ginseng. There is little if any scientific evidence that they improve performance. What evidence there is is in the form of very poorly controlled studies using limited numbers of subjects.

The vast majority of these substances provide no benefits save that gained by the placebo effect, and the bulk of their promotion relies on endorsement and testimonials by sporting celebrities. Even though they have generally been proved worthless, the mystique of these products continues to captivate almost everyone associated with sport.

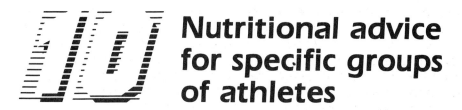

Nutritional advice for specific groups of athletes

While the information given in the previous chapters applies equally well to all athletes, there are specific groups who require special nutritional advice.

The female athlete

The nutritional needs of female athletes are not greatly dissimilar from those of their male counterparts. Both require the same nutrients and possess the same cellular mechanisms controlling the metabolic and physiological responses to exercise. Any differences that do exist between the sexes are in terms of magnitude of requirements (either needing more or less of a particular nutrient). For example, female athletes generally need less energy than males, yet require more iron.

Energy requirements

The lower energy requirements of female athletes in general can be attributed primarily to their smaller size. Not only are they lighter in weight, but relatively less of their body mass is composed of lean tissue. As women have less lean body mass and more fat than men of comparable size, they have lower energy needs for the metabolically active cells of the body. However, it should be noted that the energy requirements of a large female shot-putter weighing over 80 kg/168 lb will clearly be greater than that of the male cox of a rowing eight weighing less than 50 kg/112 lb! So, it is not possible to prescribe a particular energy requirement for a given individual, male or female.

Iron intakes

Low intakes of iron can be associated with either low energy intakes or high energy intakes (where the bulk of the energy comes from highly processed foods). This is particularly important when menstrual losses are high and the food intake is voluntarily restricted in order to maintain a low body weight.

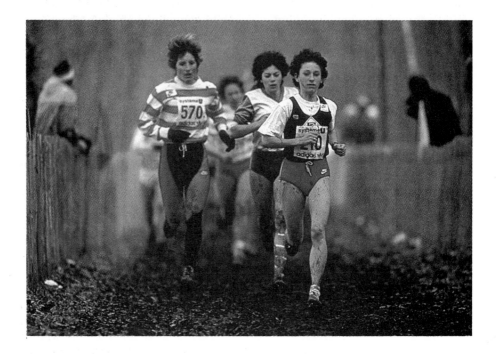

Menstrual irregularities

The restricted diet may also be a contributing factor in the development of menstrual pattern alterations in female athletes. Dysmenorrhoea (irregular periods) and amenorrhoea (complete cessation of menstrual cycle) are suprisingly commonplace amongst competitive female athletes. Women who exercise intensely often show irregularities in their menstrual cycle and even prolonged amenorrhoea: recent reports suggest that as many as 50 per cent of competitive female endurance runners and 44 per cent of professional ballet dancers suffer profound disturbances in their menstrual cycle. Sports where body weight is less important appear to have lower incidences: only 12 per cent of swimmers and cyclists report menstrual dysfunction. This may reflect the low body weights and restricted food intake associated with certain sports.

The underlying cause of this disturbance in menstrual function is unclear but it is obviously a complex psychological and physiological phenomenon involving the interaction between exercise, body weight and diet. The incidence of amenorrhoea appears related to the stress of exercise, the quantity and quality of training, the extent of weight loss, disturbances in hormonal balance, and dietary inadequacies. However, the low body weights — and lack of body fat in particular — associated with the severely restricted energy and nutrient intakes of some athletes give particular cause for concern.

Amenorrhoea is welcomed by many female athletes during the competitive season and has been generally viewed as a benign side-effect of endurance training. Yet there is recent evidence suggesting that such irregularities should be more closely examined:

- The popular suggestion that simply discontinuing training and gaining some weight will guarantee the return of fertility and a normal menstrual cycle has yet to be proven. A normal menstrual cycle may take between six months and several years to become re-established. More notably, the failure in the young adolescent to establish a normal menstrual cycle before becoming amenorrhoeic may result in particular difficulties in establishing a cycle in later life and should therefore be avoided.
- The alterations in metabolism associated with exercise-induced amenorrhoea are similar in many ways to the hormonal changes observed during the menopause. These lead to an accelerated loss of bone and the development of a condition called osteoporosis. Recent studies have shown that amenorrhoeic athletes have lower amounts of minerals (especially calcium) in their bones than normal female athletes of comparable weight, body fat and training. If this is the case, then amenorrhoeic athletes will be more prone to stress fractures and bone fragility — further studies are required to confirm this hypothesis. Simply increasing the calcium intake of such individuals per se is unlikely to resolve the problem completely especially if the underlying cause of the amenorrhoea is not detected and treated. Female athletes should be encouraged to have persistent menstrual irregularities fully examined, to avoid restricted food intakes and to consume regularly foods rich in calcium and iron.

Eating disorders

Disturbances in eating habits are often observed in young female athletes attempting to control their weight, a problem that should not be overlooked. In young gymnasts, for example, the desire to retain the comparatively masculine physique of the pre-adolescent — and associated power:weight ratio — can often be achieved through restricting growth and sexual development by limiting food intake. What starts as simply calorie counting may easily get out of hand and unfortunately this is frequently missed by coaches and parents alike.

Simple anorexia (the loss of normal appetite) is often associated with prolonged periods of caloric restriction and heavy training. While this is frequently temporary, it can easily lead to more profound disturbances. In the attempt to lower weight or maintain a very low body weight, some young female athletes find that they voluntarily restrict their intake of food considerably (often to less than 4.2 MJ/1000 kcals each day). The ensuing loss of body fat is initially associated with improvements in performance, particularly in sports such as distance running where body weight is important. This provides further incentive to continue with the restrictions in food intake. However, the severity of chronic food restriction may result in excessive reductions in body fat and deficiencies in nutrient intake, which are then reflected in an increased prevalence of injury and infection, the inability to maintain the training programme and an overall deterioration in performance.

Athletes with eating habit disorders will often deny that they are dieting despite dramatic weight loss. Other early clues of possible disturbances in eating habits are the willingness to skip meals, dislike of eating meals with others, amenorrhoea, denial of serious injuries or weight gain and depression. Such problems are not totally restricted to female athletes. Young jockeys and other athletes competing at specific weights like boxers, wrestlers and lightweight rowers, may also experience similar disturbances.

Simple anorexia should not always be directly associated with anorexia nervosa (a psychological condition characterized by a severe rejection of food) as it is frequently an intentional act whereby the female athlete is fully aware of the situation and appetite is unimpaired. This hunger in the face of deprivation often leads to eating binges followed by self-induced regurgitation and vomiting — a condition described as bulimia.

It is difficult enough in the face of an overcommitted lifestyle for the athlete to establish normal eating habits, so any additional restrictions on normal patterns of eating require closer examination and professional advice.

The young athlete

The demands placed on the body during the rapid growth and development of adolescence mean that most nutrients are required in considerably greater amounts (in proportion to body size) than in later life. The requirements for calcium and nicotinic acid are greater during adolescence than for adults

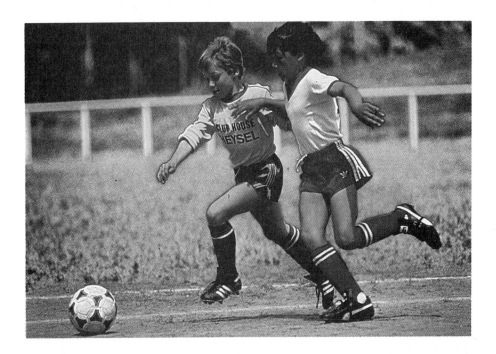

(see Appendix III, page 178). While the impact of regular training on these requirements is not clear, exercise would tend to place further demands. So it is essential that the young athlete is aware of the need for good eating habits and is actively encouraged to consume a diet rich in nutrients.

The eating habits of most children, and teenagers in particular, are known to be poor. They often skip meals or survive on 'junk food'. The lack of nutrition education in schools, coupled with the sophisticated marketing campaigns by the food industry aimed specifically at the young, often means that undesirable eating habits are established early in life and are difficult to shake off later. Young children need to be introduced to a variety of different foods, both in the home and at school, and educated in the principles of sound nutrition.

There are two particular nutritional areas that deserve attention:

● A substantial proportion of the daily intake of nutrients (of carbohydrate in particular) in the diet of many teenagers comes from highly processed food and confectionery. Consequently enforcing the total exclusion of such items from their diet can often have catastrophic effects on nutrient intake unless replaced by suitable alternatives. In many instances, excluding such foods would be comparable to putting

145

the teenager on a low-carbohydrate diet as 'junk food' often provides some 60–80 per cent of the daily carbohydrate intake of young people.
- The temperature regulating capacity of prepubescent athletes is considerably less than that of adults. They are less able to control body temperature when exercising in the heat as the sweat glands of the skin are not yet fully developed, so they are less able to cool the body by this mechanism. Young athletes are also less able to adapt to periods of prolonged sweating or acclimatize to the heat as effectively as adults as the sweat glands only possess a limited ability to produce a more dilute and copious sweat, thus conserving electrolytes. Therefore, as the young athlete is more prone to heat exhaustion than an adult athlete, considerable care should be taken when exercising in the heat and adequate hydration should be ensured.

The vegetarian and vegan athlete

The term vegetarian has several meanings. A strict vegetarian (often referred to as a vegan) uses only plant sources as food and no animal produce is eaten at all. Some vegetarians include milk, cheese and eggs (the lacto-ovo vegetarians) whilst others even eat fish and seafood, simply abstaining from meat.

The popularity of vegetarianism, in its many forms, has increased dramatically over the last decade, particularly amongst the athletic community. And while many athletes have become vegetarians and some even vegans, many have simply stopped eating red meat. This decision may have been made on moral grounds or purely to achieve a healthier diet.

Is there any harm in adopting such an approach? In nutritional terms, it is quite possible to obtain all the nutrients that may be required in sufficient quantities without eating meat. Any nutrients normally provided by meat within our diet can be obtained from other sources. For example, the use of dairy produce, such as milk and cheese, combined with the increased consumption of legumes, whole grain cereals and vegetables, will provide more than sufficient amounts of essential amino acids, vitamins and minerals. Totally excluding all animal products does, though, place an even greater dependence on the remaining foods in the diet, so if you are considering a vegetarian diet make sure you are sufficiently well educated in nutrition to be able to select the right foods. Nutritional naivety, coupled with radical alterations in eating habits (sometimes overenthusiastically pursued), can have disastrous results.

Certain nutrients may be limited in the diet of vegetarians, and vegans in particular. Iron — especially in the form that is more readily absorbed in the gut (haem–iron) — is primarily derived from animal flesh and organs (liver, kidney, red meats, game, etc). Potential deficiencies can be prevented by ensuring that the consumption of other sources of iron (such as green leafy vegetables, beans, nuts and whole grain cereals, is increased (see Chapter 8). Increasing vitamin C intake by consuming more fresh fruit and vegetables will also improve absorption of non-haem iron. Other nutrients, such as calcium and vitamin B_2 may also be limited in the diet of strict vegetarians but in these cases the addition of milk and dairy produce greatly reduces the possibility of nutritional inadequacies developing.

Despite restricting their choice of food considerably, vegans can obtain all the nutrients they require from plant sources with the exception of vitamin B_{12}. Yet surprisingly few vegans actually show signs of B_{12} deficiency which may be due to an increased awareness of the benefits of using a B_{12} supplement or possibly because the microbial contamination of food provides sufficient B_{12} to meet requirements.

Will excluding red meats and animal products from the diet improve performance? This has not been determined but there have certainly been many very successful vegetarian athletes so it does not necessarily impair performance. What is clear is that athletes who have decided to improve their eating habits (like the lacto-ovo vegetarian) are much better educated and more aware of how their diet can influence both their health and their performance. They also tend to consume a much higher proportion of their energy in the form of starchy carbohydrate consuming relatively little fat and sugar in comparison with their meat-eating counterparts. Consequently, they may find that they are able to train more effectively by ensuring adequate refuelling between training sessions (see Chapter 4).

To summarize, it would appear that radical departures from traditional habits, such as veganism, are not without their complications, but taking some steps along the path of vegetarianism may be advantageous for many athletes. The occasional serving of meat-free dishes or those incorporating only a small amount of meat and the use of lean meats and dairy produce will help to increase carbohydrate intake while keeping fats low.

The injured or retiring athlete

One of the greatest nutritional problems facing an athlete arises during the period of enforced rest that normally accompanies an injury. The considerable appetite normally associated with intense training often continues despite a dramatic and abrupt decrease in energy expenditure. Many injured athletes, who normally eat a high-energy diet, often find that their body weight increases easily during the rest period. This can often delay the return to competitive sport as the excess weight must be removed. Considerable attention should therefore be paid to ensuring that the gain in body weight

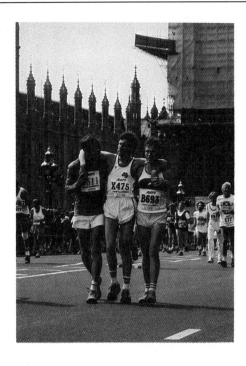

is minimal, particularly during prolonged periods of injury. Unless some other form of exercise is possible while the athlete is injured, this will mean reducing the energy intake but ensuring that the supply of protein, vitamins and minerals remains high.

The body's requirement for many vitamins and minerals, particularly vitamin C, is believed to increase following injury and infection. Inadequate supplies of such nutrients will clearly retard wound healing and tissue repair, but there is little evidence that recovery is enhanced by supplementing an already adequate diet. These needs can usually be met by the normal diet though, if the energy is restricted, it is important that the nutrient density is maintained at high levels.

In certain instances, appetite may be lost because of infection and this again will result in a reduced intake of nutrients at a time of increased requirements. This is one occasion when a single multivitamin/mineral supplement or a complete liquid meal may be warranted.

Similarly, at the end of the season or retirement, excessive increases in body fat (brought about by continued consumption of a high-energy diet when energy needs are reduced) should be avoided. The good eating habits that you pursued in the name of performance should not be ignored once you stop competing!

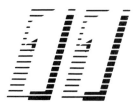 # Theory into practice

The athlete

The information contained within these pages may cause you to reconsider many long held beliefs about your diet. But before rushing in and changing your eating habits dramatically, consider each change carefully and plan accordingly.

While it is easy to change your attitudes overnight, such rapid changes to your eating habits would cause all manner of imbalances and confusion. Changes should be introduced slowly, step-by-step, ensuring that each modification is accommodated into your normal way of life with the minimum disturbance. This will ensure that you keep to your new eating habits for life.

Food diaries

To assess your own eating habits, start off by keeping a record of your present eating habits during a period of training in a food diary (see Figure 11.1). Write down everything you eat and drink from the moment you rise in the morning to when you go to bed; if you are keeping a training log already, incorporate the food diary into that. Make no attempt to modify your diet at this stage.

Ideally keep a food diary for seven days to accommodate variations in food intake, although as little as three days (including a Saturday or Sunday, ie, Thursday to Saturday or Sunday to Tuesday) may be sufficient to identify a pattern. Weigh yourself at the beginning and end of the period. Record as much information in the diary as possible:

- The type of food eaten and how much, either as a simple estimate of portion size or as an actual weight using kitchen scales. Do not forget to note how you weighed the food (ie, with skin, without skin, with bones, etc)
- The time the food was eaten, where and why it was eaten — perhaps you were hungry and it was the first food available or it was simply what you fancied at the time.

149

- Details of how your eating patterns fitted in with your training. Did you bother to prepare any food after training or was there food ready for you when you returned home?
- Details of how you felt at the time of eating, eg, 'I trained on a full stomach', or 'I felt very hungry for the hour before training', or 'I wish I hadn't eaten that meal so late last night'. This sort of analysis may help you to pinpoint areas of improvement.
- Details of drink prior to, during and after training. Were you thirsty before you started training?

The record should enable you to examine your normal pattern of eating to see how your lifestyle dictates what you eat, when, where and why. You should then ask the following questions:

- Is there room for improvement or is your diet better than you had originally thought?

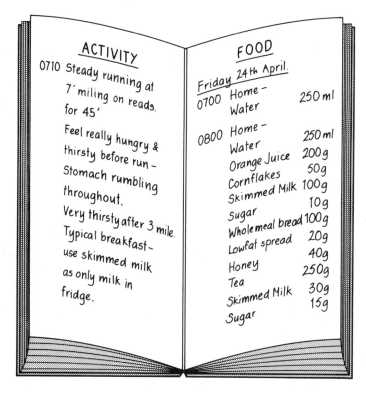

Fig.11.1 A page from a food diary.

● Are some days better than others, and is there any relationship between diet and the days when training went particularly well?
● Do you feel more tired as the week progresses?
● What foods dominate your diet and what foods are eaten occasionally? Do you survive on the same food each day or is there variety in your diet? How much starchy high-fibre foods, such as cereals, fresh vegetables and fruit, do you eat and what proportion of the foods in your diet are processed and made up of large amounts of fat or sugar?

Before making alterations to your existing eating habits, you should also consider whether there are constraints placed upon your lifestyle that may prevent you from making the necessary changes. For example, do you have any say in what you eat or do you just eat whatever is cooked for you? Can you cook? When do you eat the main meal of the day? What proportion of your meals are eaten away from home each day? Are there financial constraints on your eating habits or is it simply a case of too little time and not enough effort? Do you dislike those foods that are meant to be good for you? Unless you come to terms with such aspects of your lifestyle, even the most motivated athlete will find it difficult to make substantial long-lasting changes to his diet.

Once you have assessed your diary, gradually start to introduce the recommendations for a healthy diet mentioned in the foregone chapters and then repeat the food diary exercise six to eight weeks later. Identify where you have been successful and work on those weaker, more stubborn aspects of your diet. Having examined your eating habits in training, try the same exercise at the height of competition.

Assessing your nutrient intake

If you decide to keep a very accurate food diary (see Figure 11.1) it is possible to make an objective qualitative assessment of your nutrient intake by using food composition tables (see page 163). These tables contain analyses for most foods including packaged and processed foods: in addition, the nutritional composition of many commercial products is now included on the packaging.

The analysis will tell you the amount of energy, protein, carbohydrate, fat, fibre, vitamins, minerals in each food item. For example, 100 g of raw potato contains 75.8 g water/0.5 g sugar/20.3 g starch/2.1 g fibre and so on. Instead of using these results as a means of identifying specific deficiencies, use them to examine what contribution each item of food makes to your total intake of each nutrient over the day. For example, what items of food provide the most energy, the most carbohydrate, or vitamins? Do some

Table 11.1 Nutrient composition of the diet

Here are two typical days' food intake. The nutrient composition of each food has been determined and the relative contributions of protein, fat, carbohydrate and alcohol towards the total energy intake have been calculated.

For example, as Diet 1 provided 119 g of protein and the total intake was 14822 kJ:

each gram of protein provides 17 kJ, so

119 × 17 kJ = 2023 kJ

So protein provided

$$\frac{2023}{14822} \times 100 \quad \text{of the total energy intake} = 13.6\%$$

Diet I Nutrient composition of a traditional diet

Food	Wt (g)	Energy (kJ)	Prot (g)	Fat (g)	CHO (g)	Fibre (g)	Ca (mg)	Fe (mg)	C (mg)	B (mg)
Breakfast										
Sausage Fried	60	912	6·4	19·3	5·7	0	25	0·7	0	0
Bacon Fried	60	1110	14·7	23·3	0	0	7	0·8	0	0·2
Eggs Fried	45	275	5·5	4·9	0	0	23	0·9	0	0
Bread Fried	30	297	2·3	5·0	14·9	0·8	30	0·5	0	0·1
Lard	30	1100	0	30	0	0	0	0	0	0
Coffee	5	21	0·7	0	0·5	0	8	0·2	0	0
Milk	30	82	1·0	1·1	1·4	0	36	0	1	0
Sugar	30	504	0	0	32·0	0	1	0	0	0
Lunch										
Mars bar	45	834	2·4	8·5	29·9	0	72	0·5	0	0
Cheese	20	1680	26·0	33·5	0	0	800	0·4	0	0
Butter	100	608	0·8	16·4	0	0	3	0	0	0
White roll	80	793	6·2	1·4	39·8	2·2	80	1·4	0	0·1
Crisps	30	667	1·9	10·8	14·8	3·6	11	0·6	5	0·1
Coca-cola	285	479	0	0	29·9	0	11	0	0	0
Dinner										
Cod in batter	200	1670	39·2	20·6	15·0	0	160	1·0	0	0·1
Chips	250	2660	9·5	27·2	93·2	6·3	35	2·3	15	0·3
2 pints beer	1140	1130	2·4	0	26·2	0	90	0	0	0
TOTALS		14822	119	197·5	303·3	12·9	1392	9·3	21	0·9
% energy from	×	×	13·6	49·3	32·7 + 4·4% alcohol	×	×	×	×	×

Diet II Nutrient composition of a healthy day's intake

Food	Wt (g)	Energy (kJ)	Prot (g)	Fat (g)	CHO (g)	Fibre (g)	Ca (mg)	Fe (mg)	C (mg)	B (mg)
Breakfast										
Muesli	100	1560	13·0	7·6	66·2	7·4	200	4·6	0	0·4
Skimmed milk	250	335	8·5	0·3	12·5	0	325	0·1	4	0·1
Wholemeal toast	100	918	8·8	2·7	41·8	8·5	23	2·5	0	0·3
Low fat spread	20	301	0	8·1	0	0	0	0	0	0
Honey	50	615	0·2	0	38·2	0	2·5	0·2	0	0
Fresh orange juice	150	215	0·6	0	12·7	0	14	0·8	53	0·1
Tea	3	0	0	0	0	0	0	0	0	0
Skimmed milk	30	43	1·0	0	1·5	0	39	0	1	0
Lunch										
Wholemeal bread	100	918	8·8	2·7	41·8	8·5	23	2·5	0	0·3
Low fat spread	20	301	0	8·1	0	0	0	0	0	0
Lean ham	50	560	12·4	9·5	0	0	5	0·7	0	0·2
Tomato	25	15	0·2	0	0·7	0·4	3	0·1	5	0
Lettuce	15	5	0·1	0	0·2	0·2	3	0·1	2	0
Apple	150	294	0·5	0	17·9	2·3	6	0·5	7	0·1
Dinner										
Chicken roast	120	719	31·8	4·8	0	0	11	0·6	0	0·1
Jacket potato	200	900	5·2	5·2	50·0	5	20	1·6	20	0·2
Sweetcorn	60	195	1·7	0·3	9·7	3·4	2	0·4	2	0
Runner beans	60	61	1·4	0	2·3	2·0	16	0·5	12	0
Cauliflower	80	45	1·5	0	1·2	1·4	17	0·4	51	0·1
Tinned peaches	120	560	0·6	0	34·3	3	6	0·6	6	0
Ice cream	150	1050	5·2	11·1	34·2	0	195	0·5	1	0·1
TOTALS		9610	101·5	60·4	365	42·1	910·5	16·7	164	2·0
% energy from	×	×	17·9	21·3	60·7	×	×	×	×	×

foods provide little in the way of nutrients yet feature predominantly in the diet — eg, alcohol, sweets and chocolates? Use the tables to compare foods in terms of nutrient content and identify alternative foods that would contribute more profoundly to your diet.

Take a critical look at what you eat

First, establish the total amount of energy you consume each day, using the energy values in the food composition tables. If your weight remains constant over the food diary period (and the record is representative of your normal eating habits), your energy intake is at the correct level, ie, energy intake balances energy expenditure. If you are gaining weight, your energy intake is too high and, if you are losing weight, it is too low.

Second, determine the proportions of energy that are derived from fat, carbohydrate, protein and alcohol, express them as a percentage of the total daily intake of energy (ie, 30 per cent carbohydrate, 10 per cent fat, etc) and then compare these against the latest recommendations (see page 178). If your diet does not conform with the recommended values, look back over your food diary to see how each food contributed to the intake of each nutrient. For example, if the percentage of fat is too high, you are probably eating too many high-fat animal products. You can reduce the consumption of these foods in a number of ways: by eating smaller portions, eating them less frequently or substituting foods that are low in fat. As a general rule, your carbohydrate intake is likely to be low if you are eating too much fat, so try replacing the energy vacated by a low fat intake with more starchy high-fibre foods — thus shifting the emphasis towards carbohydrates.

Your findings should not be interpreted too rigorously without further clinical or biochemical assessment. Discuss your findings with your coach or fellow athletes. If you want more specific advice, you will need the assistance of a professional nutritionist or dietitian. Show the dietitian the dietary analysis you have conducted as this will make it much easier for the dietition to comment on your eating habits.

Do not become so concerned with your diet that you ignore other parts of your training and lifestyle that could benefit from change as well. Also be wary of trying to convert others to your new ideas before you have adopted them in full yourself and shown that they work for you. Most importantly do not expect dramatic improvements in performance overnight. These will come from adapative changes in response to training and good eating habits support this process. It will take time, maybe several years, and you must be patient. Poor dietary practices may have been detrimental to your performance in the past and you may even have underachieved in your sport as a result. But, if sound eating habits are maintained, a slow but steady improvement in performance will be achieved.

The coach

The coach has a particular responsibility to encourage sound nutritional practices and to ensure that any myths and misconceptions about nutrition do not impair the development or growth of the athlete. The coach's own understanding and beliefs will dictate many of the practices adopted by the athlete, so it is essential that the coach continues his own education (through coaching workshops, study days on nutrition or literature) to ensure his advice is correct and uptodate. He should also practise what he preaches, as there is little point in extolling the virtues of sound eating habits if your own dietary practices do not conform.

It is important not to be over enthusiastic about nutrition. Forcing new attitudes and practices upon unwilling athletes will result in conflict, resistance and poor compliance. An athlete's diet is often used as an excuse for underperformance; if performance is suddenly impaired after a change in eating habits, the latter may be blamed even though the fault lies elsewhere. This may cause the athlete to abandon new eating habits and revert to practices that prevailed prior to intervention. Moreover, the athlete may be particularly resistant to further attempts to improve his diet.

Advising the athlete

First encourage the athlete to keep a food diary as described on page 149 and then discuss the findings with them. Make yourself aware of what your athlete eats. Encourage him to complete a simple questionnaire (see page 168) to find out his nutritional beliefs and the extent of his knowledge. Identify patterns of food consumption, likes and dislikes of each athlete in your care, as these facts will be useful when on tour or at a competition away from home (see below). Discuss the eating habits of young athletes with parents or guardians, rather than the children themselves, to avoid conflict at home.

The informed coach should know where to seek professional advice, eg, from a dietitian or doctor, but he may be able to help the athlete to improve his diet in specific areas:

- Erratic meals and eating habits (see page 151)
- Very low carbohydrate intakes (see page 75)
- Excessive weight restriction and hyponutrition in young girls (see page 144)
- Controlled weight loss or making weight (see page 109)
- Gaining weight (see page 118)
- Fluid balance during training and competition (see page 86)

155

- Use of vitamin/mineral supplements and ergogenic aids (see page 121)
- Preparation for competition (see page 96)
- Purchase and preparation of food (see page 151).

Competitions

When taking individual or team athletes to competitions away from home, you will have to ensure that the different eating habits of everyone on the tour are accommodated both during the training period and during the competition itself, otherwise performance can be impaired. Do not insist that every member of the team eats the same meals or follows the same pre-match/pre-competition preparation — wherever possible try to accommodate personal requirements. If travelling abroad:

1) Check out feeding arrangements in advance (before travelling)
2) Take tinned or packeted food from your home country as a backup supply.

Educating your athletes about nutrition

There are a number of ways to introduce nutrition to the performer. For example, arrange a discussion on nutrition at a club evening or at training camp — an ideal way to fill the hour after a meal when you cannot train. This could take the form of an informal discussion led by yourself, the coach, or an invited speaker, such as the dietitian from the local hospital. A tape–slide presentation or video on sports nutrition will help to liven up the discussion. Many manufacturers of commercial nutrition products also offer an advisory service and some will even produce a speaker for a club evening, but always bear in mind that the speaker may be biased towards his own product. When inviting such speakers to the club, the coach should be in a position to challenge or refute statements that appear misleading, contentious or biased.

Alternatively arrange a nutrition quiz between two or more teams. The questions can be tailored to suit the age and knowledge of the athletes (see nutritional questionnaire, page 168). Discussion of the correct answers after each question or at the end of the session will help to educate the athletes in a comparatively painless and enjoyable fashion.

Finally why not provide a meal during a club evening to illustrate just what you mean by healthy eating. This will also allow you to introduce foods which many young athletes may never have eaten at home.

156

Questions and answers

During a team sport such as rugby or soccer, there is little opportunity for players to take fluid once the game is in progress. Is it sensible to discourage players from drinking during training in order to condition them to the effects of dehydration during a game?

Certainly not! Every time your players train, they are at risk from dehydration which will not only affect their performance but also their well being (see page 86). Forcing them to train without fluids will increase the risk of hyperthermia and limit their capacity to train. This is particularly important when training in a warm environment — during the summer months, training inside gyms or when abroad. If anything, you should condition your players to take fluid (preferably water) little and often throughout a training session so they get used to exercising with fluid in their stomachs. During a game or competition, players should take fluid at every opportunity, for example during natural stoppages and breaks for injury, and not just at half time. Each player could have their own container eg, a cyclist's water bottle.

I am a heavy-weight boxer and need to put on weight as muscle but I cannot afford to buy steaks, eggs, or expensive protein supplements. What should I eat?

The only way to increase your muscle mass is through a planned and systematic programme of intensive resistance or weight training. Consuming large amounts of protein on top of your normal diet will do little to increase the rate at which muscle is gained (see page 118); it can actually limit your ability to train thereby reducing your chances of increasing muscle mass. Consuming large amounts of protein will leave you with little appetite or desire to eat the all important starchy carbohydrate foods necessary to refuel your energy reserves between training sessions (see page 74). Inadequate glycogen repletion means an impaired ability to train. Instead of eating more protein, you should concentrate on ensuring that your diet contains food (such as cereals and legumes) that are rich in carbohydrate, fibre, minerals and vitamins as well as protein — and carbohydrate-rich foods are often cheaper to buy if budget is a problem.

I am a coach taking a team of cyclists abroad to compete in a tournament later this year. What can I do in advance to make sure that their performance does not suffer from poor nutrition while we are away?

The most important thing to remember is to leave nothing to chance and always prepare yourself fully before leaving for the competition. Research

157

the type of food that will be available both at your hotel and at the cycling stadium, not forgetting food during the journey to and from the stadium if it is a long drive. Is the type and quality of food comparable to home standards and can the cyclists eat meals at the times they are used to eating — particularly on the days of competition? Discuss your requirements with the organizers of the event or hotel in advance. Ensure that personal dislikes do not appear on the menu too frequently. If any food is likely to cause gut disturbances or if the water is unsuitable for drinking from the tap, make sure everybody in the party is aware of these facts. Take a supply of confectionery, breakfast cereals and canned food with you as these are particularly useful if one of the team loses his appetite. Try to ensure that normal eating habits are disrupted as little as possible.

As a tennis player, I compete throughout the season with very little time to recover between matches. What can I do to help myself to recover more effectively?

Every time you play a tennis game you make substantial inroads into your glycogen stores. The longer or harder the match, the greater the extent of glycogen depletion (see page 74) and the longer it will take to refuel fully those stores. Similarly, you will become dehydrated each time you play. You must try to offset the progressive depletion of muscle glycogen and dehydration by ensuring that you take adequate carbohydrate and fluids in your diet at all times (see page 86). You should offset dehydration by drinking before, during and after the game and start the carbohydrate refuelling process as soon after the game as possible.

If, despite eating a diet rich in carbohydrates and other nutrients sufficient to maintain your normal competition weight, you still feel tired, then you must rest for longer periods between competitions to allow your body time to recover.

Are oranges the best refreshment to take at half-time?

While oranges are refreshing and will cleanse the palate, they do little to replace vital fluids lost during exercise. The electrolytes and vitamin C gained from a piece of orange are of little immediate value and, in the limited time available at half-time, it is better to drink water or some form of dilute drink in order to rehydrate. If the weather is particularly cold, you may prefer something warm, like weak tea.

Are glucose tablets, sugary drinks and confectionery good sources of extra energy, especially when taken just before exercise?

Many athletes are under the misconception that the consumption of sugar-rich foods and drinks just before the start of a race or game will help to provide them with a much-needed burst of energy. However, glucose (or any disaccharide equivalent to a confectionery bar) taken within 30–60 minutes prior to playing most sports can actually impair performance for the following reasons:

- Although the glucose is rapidly absorbed into the blood from the intestine, little of it is available for use by the working muscle. Instead, the rapid increase in blood glucose concentration (hyperglycaemia) will cause the release of insulin from the pancreas (a hormone for controlling blood glucose levels).
- If exercise is initiated with high insulin levels, glucose is rapidly transported into the body cells, resulting in an equally rapid fall in blood glucose beyond normal resting values (known as rebound hypoglycaemia).
- As a result, the supply of glucose to the brain (so vital for normal functioning) will be reduced, often causing confusion, disorientation and nausea.
- In addition, elevated insulin levels will inhibit fat mobilization, placing an even greater dependency on the limited reserves of glycogen.
- Finally, a high concentration of glucose in the stomach will limit fluid absorption, precipitating more pronounced dehydration.

To avoid such an upset, it is advisable not to take glucose tablets, sugary drinks or confectionery within 30 minutes of the start of of a race. It would be much better to save your confectionery until immediately after the race, when you start your refuelling process.

Should athletes drink alcohol?

A few studies have shown that alcohol, when used as an ergogenic aid immediately prior to or during competition, may improve performance in certain activities. But most evidence suggests that even small amounts of alcohol taken during exercise have a deleterious effect on sporting performance.

In contrast, there is little evidence to suggest that a **moderate** consumption of alcohol in a social environment will impair performance. It should not be overlooked that many people play sport just to enjoy the

159

company of others socially after the game — it doesn't make them any less of an athlete.

However, there are two reasons for discouraging the consumption of alcohol by the competitive athlete, even at a social level:

- Firstly, alcohol is a potent diuretic and will promote dehydration. Any athlete training regularly in the morning would be advised to limit alcohol consumption the evening before to ensure that he does not start training in a dehydrated condition. Moreover, after consuming alcohol, the capacity of the liver to maintain blood glucose levels by gluconeogenesis is severely limited, prolonged training with a hang-over may precipitate hypoglycaemia.
- Secondly, although alcoholic drinks are high in energy (in the form of alcohol not sugar), little of the energy is available to the working muscle during exercise; they are also low in essential nutrients, so alcohol takes up nutrient space in the diet that could be used more effectively. The contribution made by alcohol to the total energy intake of the average adult is around 6 per cent, yet it can provide as much as 10–20 per cent, even in people who believe that they drink modestly. Finally, like any drug, the excessive use of or reliance upon, alcohol will obviously have long term consequences, not only on performance but also on the health of the athlete.

My daughter is about to take part in a 24-hour badminton marathon. What should she eat before and during the marathon?

First, ensure that she gets to the start of the event adequately recovered from the training period, ie, with at least normal glycogen and fluid reserves. This can be achieved by ensuring that her normal diet over the months leading up to the event is rich in starchy carbohydrates. By tapering the training over the final week and maintaining an emphasis on starchy foods you will ensure that normal glycogen reserves are re-established. Consuming sugary foods in addition to starchy foods over the last few days will promote refuelling. Throughout training, she should have conditioned her body to take fluid in between games and her fluid intake should be increased over the final week as well, particularly the day before the event and on the day of the event.

Second, ensure that high-carbohydrate starchy foods, such as sand-wiches and muesli bars, and fluids, especially water, are available throughout the event. Similarly hot drinks containing some sugar, and confectionery should also be available. Commercial energy drinks may be helpful, but all these foods should have been tried and tested during the training period, not eaten or drunk for the first time at the event. Rather than preselect just one or two foods for the event, bring along a large variety of food and let her choose. Remember that no two players will respond the same way to the event and that the likes and dislikes of your daughter may change as the event progresses.

This advice is equally applicable to anybody participating in an event that lasts for one or several days.

Whenever I compete in endurance events, I experience severe abdominal pains and get acute diarrhoea either during or immediately after the race. Yet this rarely happens during training runs. This condition has forced me to retire from several major races. Is there anything I can do?

This condition, often referred to as 'runners' trots' is extremely common and can have disastrous consequences. Interestingly it does not always appear to be related to diet or the overconsumption of fluids while running — although the latter would certainly result in similar symptoms as well as vomiting and nausea. A more likely explanation appears to be related to the changes in blood flow and nervous stimulation of the intestine. During the race you will probably be running harder and longer than you would during a training session: the symptoms develop because your intestine is contracting vigorously against itself. Certain drugs, that cause the muscles of the intestine to relax, may help but these drugs should only be used on the advice of your doctor.

I want to get fit and lose weight, so I have taken up aerobics and have put myself on a weight-reducing diet. However, I just cannot seem to stick to my diet and keep training at the same time. What sort of diet should I be following?

The inability to maintain a heavy training programme and a weight-reducing diet at the same time usually means that you are expending more energy than you are taking in, ie, you have reduced your energy intake by too much. Your glycogen stores are not being sufficiently replenished between training sessions, so you are doing aerobics on 'empty muscles' (see page 74). Try not to over-restrict your energy intake; rather than eat, for example, 2–4 MJ each day, eat around 6–8 MJ and increase energy expenditure. It is a fact that, by combining exercise with dieting, you do not need to restrict your diet by so much. Remember to reduce fat in your diet and ensure you eat plenty of starchy high-fibre foods instead (see page 113).

I am a keen badminton player and an insulin-dependent diabetic. In order to maintain control, I have to keep a careful eye on my carbohydrate intake. Should I follow the advice to eat more carbohydrate in training?

The amount of carbohydrate that should be eaten by a diabetic has been debated for many years. Contrary to the old dogma that diabetics should restrict their consumption of carbohydrate and derive energy from fats and proteins, there is now considerable evidence to suggest that improved carbohydrate tolerance and diminished requirements for insulin results from a diet rich in starchy, high-fibre carbohydrate and low in fat — the exact opposite. This more liberal approach to diet does not mean diabetics can eat what they like — sugar intakes must be restricted to prevent episodes of hyperglycaemia, and the overall energy intake should be controlled to maintain a desirable body weight.

As a result the general advice offered in this book applies equally well to the diabetic athlete as to any other athlete. However, any alterations in carbohydrate intake by a diabetic athlete should only be considered after discussing intentions with his or her diabetologist or dietitian.

Recommended reading list

Textbooks on nutrition and physiology

1. R Passmore and M A Eastwood **Human Nutrition and Dietetics** (8th edition) (Churchill Livingstone, Edinburgh 1986)
2. Ministry of Agriculture, Fisheries and Foods **Manual of Nutrition** (9th edition) (Impression, 1985)
3. British Dietetic Association **The Great British Diet** (Century, London 1985)
4. M J Gibney **Nutrition, Diet and Health** (Cambridge University Press 1986)
5. A Maryon-Davies and J Thomas **Diet 2000** (Pan Books, London 1984)
6. V Katch and W D McArdle **Nutrition, Weight Control and Exercise** (Houghton Mifflin 1982)
7. A Bender **Health or Hoax?** (Elvendon Press 1986)

Textbooks on exercise physiology and biochemistry

1. E Fox **Sport Physiology** (W B Saunders 1984)
2. G Brookes and E Fahey **Exercise Physiology** (Wiley 1984)
3. E Newsholme and T Leech **The Runner** (W J Meagher, 1983)
4. D Costill 'A Scientific Approach to Distance Running' **(Track and Field News 1979)**
5. W D McArdle, F I Katch and V L Katch **Exercise Physiology — Energy, Nutrition and Human Performance** (2nd Edition) (Lea and Febiger 1986)
6. P O Åstrand and K Rodahl **Textbook of Work Physiology** (2nd edition) (McGraw Hill 1986)
7. D R Lamb **Physiology of Exercise** (MacMillan 1984)

Textbooks on sports nutrition

1. M H Williams **Nutritional Aspects of Human Physical and Athletic Performance** (2nd edition) (Thomas 1985)
2. A L Hecker (Editor) **Nutritional Aspects of Exercise — Clinics in Sports Medicine** Vol 3, No 3 (W B Saunders 1984)
3. D H Shrimpton and P Berry-Ottaway (Editors) **Nutrition in Sport — Proceedings of the National Symposium** (Shaklee U K, 1986)
4. P Berry-Ottaway and K Hargin **Food for Sport — A Handbook of Sports Nutrition** (Resource Publications, Cambridge 1985)

Food composition tables

1. A Paul and D A T Southgate (Editors) McCance & Widdowson's **The Composition of Foods** (4th edition) (HMSO 1978)
2. B K Watt and A L Merrill **The Composition of Foods — Raw, Processed and Prepared, Handbook 8** (US Department of Agriculture, Washington DC 1963).

Sports nutrition references

GENERAL

American Dietetic Association (1980). Nutrition and physical fitness — a statement by the A.D.A. Am Diet Assoc 76 437–443.

Brotherhood J.R. (1984). Nutrition and sports performance. Sports Med. 1 350–389.

K.A. Kirsch & H. von Ameln (1981). Feeding patterns of endurance athletes. Eur J Appl Physiol 47 197–208.

Wootton S.A. (1986). Eating habits and nutritional knowledge of British athletes and coaches. In: Procedings of National Symposium on Nutrition in Sport. Ed: D. Shrimpton & P. Berry Ottaway. Shaklee UK. pp 64–75.

GLYCOGEN DEPLETION

D.L. Costill, P.D. Gollnick. E.D. Jansson, B. Saltin & E.M. Stein (1973). Glycogen depletion pattern in human muscle fibres during distance running. Acta physiol scand 89, 374–383.

P.D. Gollnick, K. Piehl & B. Saltin (974). Selective glycogen depletion pattern in human muscle fibres after exercise of varying intensity and at varying pedalling rates. J Physiol 241, 45–57.

I. Jacobs, N. Westlin, J. Karlsson, M. Rasmusson & B. Houghton (1982). Muscle glycogen and diet in elite soccer players. Eur J Appl Physiol 48, 297–302.

B. Saltin (1973). Metabolic fundamentals in exercise. Med Sci Sports 5 (3) 137–146.

R.C. Hickson, M.J. Rennie, R.K. Conlee, W.W. Winder & J.O. Holloszy (1977). Effects of increased plasma fatty acids on glycogen utilisation and endurance. J Appl Physiol 43, 829–833.

GLYCOGEN REPLETION

K. Piehl (1974). Time course for refilling of glycogen stores in human muscle fibres following exercise-induced glycogen depletion. Acta physiol scand 90, 297–302.

J.D. MacDougall, G.R. Ward, D.G. Sale & J.R. Sutton (1977). Muscle glycogen repletion after high-intensity intermittent exercise. J Appl Physiol REEP 42 (2) 129–132.

Costill D.L., Sherman W.M., Fink W.J., Maresh C., Witten M. & Miller J.M. (1981). The role of dietary carbohydrates in muscle glycogen resynthesis after strenuous running. Am J Clin Nutr 34 1831–1836.

Sherman W.M., Costill D.L., Fink W.J., Armstrong L.E., Hagerman F.C. & Murray T.M. (1983). The marathon: recovery from acute biochemical alterations. In: Biochemistry of Exercise, Int Series on Sports Sciences vol 13. pp 312–317. Ed. H.G. Knuttgen, J.A. Vogel & J.R. Poortmans. Human Kinetic Publishers, Champaign.

Sherman W.M., Costill D.L., Fink W.J. & Miller J.M. (1981). Effect of exercise-diet manipulation on muscle glycogen and its subsequent utilisation during performance. Int J Sports Med 2, 114–118.

GLYCOGEN LEVELS AND PERFORMANCE

J. Karlsson & B. Saltin (1971). Diet, muscle glycogen and endurance performance. J Appl Physiol 31 (2) 203–206.

E. Hultman & J. Bergstrom (1967). Muscle glycogen synthesis in relation to diet studied in normal subjects. Acta medica scand 182, 109–117.

P.D. Gollnick, K. Piehl, C.W. Saubert, R.B. Armstrong & B. Saltin (1972). Diet, exercise and glycogen changes in human muscle fibres. J Appl Physiol 33 (4) 421–425.

M. Jette, O. Pelletier, L. Parker & J. Thoden (1978). The nutritional and metabolic effects of a carbohydrate-rich diet in a glycogen supercompensation training regimen. Am J Clin Nutr 31, 2140–2148.

I. Jacobs, P. Kaiser & P. Tesch (1981). Muscle strength and fatigue after selective glycogen depletion in human skeletal muscle fibres. Eur J Appl Physiol 46, 47–53.

R.J. Maughan & D.C. Poole (1981). The effects of a glycogen-loading regimen on the capacity to perform anaerobic exercise. Eur J Appl Physiol 46, 211–219.

Wootton S.A. & Williams C. (1984). Influence of carbohydrate-status on performance during maximal exercise. Int J Sports Med 5, 126–127.

CARBOHYDRATE-FEEDING ON PERFORMANCE

C. Foster, D.L. Costill & W.J. Fink (1979). Effects of pre-exercise feedings on endurance performance. Med Sci Sports Ex 11 (1) 1–5.

J.L. Ivy, D.L. Costill, W.J. Fink & R.W. Lower (1979). Influence of caffeine and carbohydrate feedings on endurance performance. Med Sci Sports 11 (1) 6–11.

D.L. Costill, E. Coyle, G. Dalsky, W. Evans, W. Fink & D. Hoopes (1977). Effects of elevated plasma FFA and insulin on muscle glycogen usage during exercise. J Appl Physiol REEP 43 695–699.

A.V. Koivisto, S. Karonen & E. Nikkila (1981). Carbohydrate ingestion before exercise: comparison of glucose, fructose and sweet placebo. J Appl Physiol REEP 51 (4) 783–787.

D.L. Costill, A. Bennett, G. Branam & D. Eddy (1973). Glucose ingestion at rest and during prolonged exercise. J Appl Physiol 34 (6) 764–769.

A. Bonen, S.A. Malcolm, R.D. Kilgour, K.P. MacIntyre & A.N. Belcastro (1981). Glucose ingestion before and during intense exercise. J Appl Physiol REEP 50 (4) 766–771.

J.L. Ivy, W. Miller, V. Dover, L.G. Goodyear, W.M. Sherman, S. Farrell & H. Williams (1983). Endurance improved by ingestion of glucose polymer supplement. Med Sci Sports & Ex 15 466–471.

M. Hargreaves, D.L. Costill, A. Coggan, W.J. Fink & I. Nishibata (1984). Carbohydrate feedings on muscle glycogen utilisation and exercise performance. Med Sci Sports Ex 16 219–222.

Coyle E.F., Hagberg J.M., Hurley B.F., Martin W.H., Ehsani A.A. & Holloszy J.D. (1983). Carbohydrate feeding during prolonged continuous exercise can delay fatigue. J Appl Physiol 55, 230–235.

BODY WEIGHT AND COMPOSITION

Wilmore J.H. (1982). Body composition and athletic performance. In: Nutrition & Athletic performance. Ed: W. Haskell, J. Scala & J. Whittam. Bull Publishing Co., Palo Alto. pp 158–175.

Buskirk E.R. & Mendez J. (1984). Sports science and body composition analysis: emphasis on cell and muscle mass. Med & Science in Sports & Ex 16, 584–593.

Tipton C.M. (1982). Consequences of rapid weight loss. In: Nutrition & Athletic performance. Ed: W. Haskell, J. Scala & J. Whittam. Bull Publishing Co., Palo Alto. pp 176–197.

M.E. Houston, D.A. Marrin, H.J. Green & J.A. Thomson (1981). The effect of rapid weight loss on physiological functions in wrestlers. Physician & Sports Med 9 (11) 73–78.

Smith N.A. (1984). Weight control in the athlete. In: Nutritional Aspects of Exercise. Clinics in Sports Medicine. pp 693–704. Ed. A.L. Hecker. W.B. Saunders Co., Philadelphia.

Marcus R., Cann C., Madvig P. et al (1985). Menstrual function and bone mass in elite women distance runners: endocrine and metabolic features. Ann Int Med 102, 158–163.

Deuster P.A., Kyle S.B., Moser P.B. et al (1986). Nutritional survey of highly trained women runners. Am J Clin Nutr 44, 954–962.

FLUID INTAKE

D.L. Costill & B. Saltin (1974). Factors limiting gastric emptying during rest and exercise. J Appl Physiol 37 (5) 679–683.

K.E. Olsson & B. Saltin (1971). Diet and fluids in training and competition. Scand J Rehab Med 3 31–38.

Costill D.L. & Miller J.M. (1980). Carbohydrate and fluid balance. Int J Sports Med 1 2–9.

Cade R., Spooner G., Sclein E, Pickering M. & Dean R. (1972). Effect of fluid, electrolyte and glucose replacement during exercise on performance, body composition, rate of sweat loss and compositional changes of extracellular fluid. J Sports Med 12, 150–156,

Coyle E.F., Costill D.L., Fink W.J. & Hooper D.G. (1978). Gastric emptying rates for selected athletic drinks. Research Quarterly 49, 119–125.

Maughan R.J. (1985). Fluid and electrolyte balance in prolonged exercise. Nutr Bull 10, 28–35.

PROTEIN METABOLISM

Lemon P.W.R. & Nagle F.J. (1981). Effects of exercise on protein and amino acid metabolism. Med & Science in Sports & Ex 13, 141–149.

Laurent G.J. & Millward D.J. (1980). Protein turnover during skeletal muscle hypertrophy. Fed Proc 29, 42–47.

Dohm G.L. (1986). Protein as a fuel for exercise. In: Exercise & Sports Science Reviews, Vol 14. Ed: K.B. Pandolf. Macmillan, New York. pp 143–173.

VITAMINS AND MINERALS

A.C. Grandjean (1983). Vitamins, diet and the athlete. Clinics in Sports Med 2 (1) 105–114.

Bruce A., Ekblom B. & Nilsson I. (1985). The effect of vitamin and mineral supplements and health foods on physical endurance and performance. Proc Nutr Soc 44 283–295.

Williams M.H. (1984). Vitamin and mineral supplements to athletes: do they help?. In: Nutritional Aspects of Exercise. Clinics in Sports Medicine. Ed. A.L. Hecker. W.B. Saunders Co., Philadelphia. pp 623–638.

J. Kuel, E. Jakob, A. Berg, H–H. Dickhuth, M. Lehmann & G. Huber (1986). Performance in relation to vitamins, irons and sports anaemia. In: Procedings of National Symposium on Nutrition in Sport. Ed: D. Shrimpton & P. Berry Ottaway. Shaklee UK. pp 24–45.

Appendix I

Self-assessment nutritional knowledge questionnaire

Indicate whether you feel that the following statements are either true (T) or false (F). If you are uncertain of the answer, indicate that you are not sure (NS). Remember that this quiz is for your own benefit — it is intended to identify those areas that you understand (correct answers), those areas where you are uncertain (not sure answers) and particularly those areas where you think you know the answer but you are actually incorrect (wrong answers). Page numbers have been given after each answer for you to refer to for the correct answer in the text.

Questions

1. Weight for weight, starchy foods such as bread and potatoes contain the same amount of energy as dairy produce.

2. When you lose weight by rapid dieting, eg, 6–8 lbs a week, very little of this weight loss is fat.

3. Adding bran to your normal diet is not a good way of obtaining a high fibre diet.

4. It does not matter how much fat is in your diet as long as it is polyunsaturated.

5. Weight for weight, margarine contains the same amount of energy as butter.

6. It is the amount of sugar in an alcoholic drink that determines its energy content.

7. Fat people always eat large amounts of food.

8. Brown sugar is better for you than white sugar.

9. The body can convert fat to carbohydrate when the stores of glycogen are low.

10. A 2400 kcal diet is the same as a 10 MJ diet.

11. You should always start the day with a cooked breakfast.

168

12. Apart from eating more food, athletes do not need to eat any differently from non-athletes.

13. In order to put on muscle, you need to eat more protein than usual.

14. Vegetable sources of protein do not contain any of the essential amino acids found in animal proteins.

15. Athletes need vitamin and mineral supplements as they use more during prolonged vigorous activity.

16. During prolonged exercise, you start off by using carbohydrate alone as a fuel then switch over to fat once your glycogen stores are depleted.

17. Sugar solutions and dextrose tablets are a good way of providing extra energy during exercise.

18. The rate at which the body refuels its glycogen stores is primarily influenced by diet.

19. As long as you eat plenty of carbohydrate, you can always fully replenish your glycogen stores within 24 hours.

20. Only endurance athletes need to eat large amounts of carbohydrate.

21. The time to start drinking fluid during exercise is when you feel thirsty.

22. Athletes need to add salt to their food in order to replace the salt lost through sweating.

23. There is no harm in taking large amounts of any vitamin — the excess simply passes straight through your body.

24. If you eat more wholemeal bread and potatoes, your intake of protein, vitamins and minerals will also increase.

25. Athletes should never eat confectionery.

Answers

1: F (see page 25)
2: T (see page 111)
3: T (see page 20)
4: F (see page 18)
5: T (see page 9)
6: F (see page 21)
7: F (see page 109)
8: F (see page 20)
9: F (see page 74)

10: T (see page 24)
11: F (see page 82)
12: T (see page 81)
13: F (see page 118)
14: F (see page 13)
15: F (see page 124)
16: F (see page 55)
17: F (see page 159)
18: T (see page 74)

19: F (see page 74)
20: F (see page 83)
21: F (see page 92)
22: F (see page 92)
23: F (see page 124)
24: T (see page 78)
25: F (see page 80)

Appendix II

American College of Sports Medicine position statement on prevention of heat injuries during distance running

The Purpose of this Position Statement is:
  (a) To alert local, national and international sponsors of distance running events of the health hazards of heat injury during distance running, and
  (b) To inform said sponsors of injury preventive actions that may reduce the frequency of this type of injury.
  The recommendations address only the manner in which distance running sports activities may be conducted to further reduce incidence of heat injury among normal athletes conditioned to participate in distance running. **The recommendations are advisory only**.
  Recommendations concerning the ingested quantity and content of fluid are merely a partial preventive to heat injury. The physiology of each individual athlete varies; strict compliance with these recommendations and the current rules governing distance running may not reduce the incidence of heat injuries among those so inclined to such injury.

Research findings

Based on research findings and current rules governing distance running competition, it is the position of the American College of Sports Medicine that:

1. Distance races (> 16 km or 10 miles) should **not** be conducted when the wet bulb temperature — globe temperature (adapted from Minard, D. Prevention of heat casualities in Marine Corps recruits. Milit. Med. 126:261, 1961. WB-GT = 0.7 [WBT] +0.2 [GT] + 0.1 [DBT]) exceeds 28°C (82.4°F).
2. During periods of the year, when the daylight dry bulb temperature often exceeds 27°C (80°F), distance races should be conducted before 9:00 A.M. or after 4:00 P.M.
3. It is the responsibility of the race sponsors to provide fluids which contain small amounts of sugar (less than 2.5 g glucose per 100 ml of water) and electrolytes (less than 10 mEq sodium and 5 mEq potassium per liter of solution).
4. Runners should be encouraged to frequently ingest fluids during competition

170

and to consume 400–500 ml (13–17 oz) of fluid 10–15 minutes before competition.

5. Rules prohibiting the administration of fluids during the first 10 kilometers (6.2 miles) of a marathon race should be amended to permit fluid ingestion at frequent intervals along the race course. In light of the high sweat rates and body temperatures during distance running in the heat, race sponsors should provide "water stations" at 3–4 kilometer (2–2.5 mile) intervals for all races of 16 kilometers (10 miles) or more.

6. Runners should be instructed in how to recognize the early warning symptoms that precede heat injury. Recognition of symptoms, cessation of running, and proper treatment can prevent heat injury. Early warning symptoms include the following: piloerection on chest and upper arms, chilling, throbbing, pressure in the chest, unsteadiness, nausea, and dry throat.

7. Race sponsors should make prior arrangements with medical personnel for the care of cases of heat injury. Responsible and informed personnel should supervise each "feeding station". Organizational personnel should reserve the right to stop runners who exhibit clear signs of heat stroke or heat exhaustion.

It is the position of the American College of Sports Medicine that policies established by local, national, and international sponsors of distance running events should adhere to these guidelines. Failure to adhere to these guidelines may jeopardize the health of competitors through heat injury.

Source: Med Sci Sports 7 (1) vii–viii 1975

American College of Sports Medicine position statement on weight loss in wrestlers

It is the position of the American College of Sports Medicine that the potential health hazards created by the procedures used to "make weight" by wrestlers can be eliminated if state and national organizations will:

1. Assess the body composition of each wrestler several weeks in advance of the competitive season. Individuals with a fat content less than five percent of their certified body weight should receive medical clearance before being allowed to compete.

2. Emphasize the fact that the daily calorie requirements of wrestlers should be obtained from a balanced diet and determined on the basis of age, body surface area, growth and physical activity levels. The minimal calorie needs of wrestlers in high schools and colleges will range from 1200 to 2400 kcal/day; therefore, it is the responsibility of coaches, school officials, physicians and parents to discourage wrestlers from securing less than their minimal needs without prior medical approval.

3. Discourage the practice of fluid deprivation and dehydration. This can be accomplished by:

(a) Educating the coaches and wrestlers on the physiological consequences and medical complications that can occur as a result of these practices.

(b) Prohibiting the single or combined use of rubber suits, steam rooms, hot boxes, saunas, laxatives, and diuretics to "make weight".

(c) Scheduling weigh-ins just prior to competition.
(d) Scheduling more official weigh-ins between team matches.
4. Permit more participants/team to compete in those weight classes (119–145 pounds) which have the highest percentages of wrestlers certified for competition.
5. Standardize regulations concerning the eligibility rules at championship tournaments so that individuals can only participate in those weight classes in which they had the highest frequencies of matches throughout the season.
6. Encourage local and county organizations to systematically collect data on the hydration state of wrestlers and its relationship to growth and development.

Source: Med Sci Sports 8 (2) xi–xiii (1976)

American College of Sports Medicine position statement on the use and abuse of anabolic-androgenic steroids in sports

Based on a comprehensive survey of the world literature and a careful analysis of the claims made for and against the efficacy of anabolic-androgenic steroids in improving human physical performance, it is the position of the American College of Sports Medicine that:

1. The administration of anabolic-androgenic steroids to healthy humans below age 50 in medically approved therapeutic doses often does not of itself bring about any significant improvements in strength, aerobic endurance, lean body mass, or body weight.
2. There is no conclusive scientific evidence that extremely large doses of anabolic-androgenic steroids either aid or hinder athletic performance.
3. The prolonged use of oral anabolic-androgenic steroids (C_{17} alkylated derivatives of testosterone) has resulted in liver disorders in some persons. Some of these disorders are apparently reversible with the cessation of drug usage, but others are not.
4. The administration of anabolic-androgenic steroids to male humans may result in a decrease in testicular size and function and a decrease in sperm production. Although these effects appear to be reversible when small doses of steroids are used for short periods of time, the reversibility of the effects of large doses over extended periods of time is unclear.
5. Serious and continuing effort should be made to educate male and female athletes, coaches, physical educators, physicians, trainers, and the general public regarding the inconsistent effects of anabolic-androgenic steroids on improvement of human physical performance and the potential dangers of taking certain forms of these substances, especially in large doses, for prolonged periods.

Source: Med Sci Sports 9 (4) xi–xiii (1977)

American College of Sports Medicine position statement on the recommended quantity and quality of exercise for developing and maintaining fitness in healthy adults

Increasing numbers of persons are becoming involved in endurance training activities and thus, the need for guidelines for exercise prescription is apparent.

Based on the existing evidence concerning exercise prescription for healthy adults and the need for guidelines, the American College of Sports Medicine makes the following recommendations for the quantity and quality of training for developing and maintaining cardiorespiratory fitness and body composition in the healthy adult:

1. Frequency of training: 3 to 5 days per week.
2. Intensity of training: 60 per cent to 90 per cent of maximum heart rate reserve or, 50 per cent to 85 per cent of maximum oxygen uptake ($\dot{V}O_2$max).
3. Duration of training: 15–60 minutes of continuous aerobic activity. Duration is dependent on the intensity of the activity, thus lower intensity activity should be conducted over a longer period of time. Because of the importance of the 'total fitness' effect and the fact that it is more readily attained in longer duration programs, and because of the potential hazards and compliance problems associated with high intensity activity, lower to moderate intensity activity of longer duration is recommended for the nonathletic adult.
4. Mode of activity: Any activity that uses large muscle groups, that can be maintained continuously, and is rhythmical and aerobic in nature (eg, running-jogging, walking-hiking, swimming, skating, bicycling, rowing, cross-country skiing, rope skipping, and various endurance game activities).

Source: Med Sci Sports (10) 3 vii–ix 1978

American College of Sports Medicine position statement on the use of alcohol in sports

Based upon a comprehensive analysis of the available research relative to the effects of alcohol upon human physical performance, it is the position of the American College of Sports Medicine that:

1. The acute ingestion of alcohol can exert a deleterious effect upon a wide variety of psychomotor skills such as reaction time, hand-eye coordination, accuracy, balance, and complex coordination.
2. Acute ingestion of alcohol will not substantially influence metabolic or physiological functions essential to physical performance such as energy metabolism, maximal oxygen consumption ($\dot{V}O_2$max), heart rate, stroke volume, cardiac output, muscle blood flow, arteriovenous oxygen difference, or respiratory dynamics. Alcohol consumption may impair body temperature regulation during prolonged exercise in a cold environment.
3. Acute alcohol ingestion will not improve and may decrease strength, power,

local muscular endurance, speed, and cardiovascular endurance.

4. Alcohol is the most abused drug in the United States and is a major contributing factor to accidents and their consequences. Also, it has been documented widely that prolonged excessive alcohol consumption can elicit pathological changes in the liver, heart, brain, and muscle, which can lead to disability and death.

5. Serious and continuing efforts should be made to educate athletes, coaches, health and physical educators, physicians, trainers, the sports media, and the general public regrding the effects of acute alcohol ingestion upon human physical performance and on the potential acute and chronic problems of excessive alcohol consumption.

Source: Med Sci Sports 14 (6) ix–xi 1982

American College of Sports Medicine position statement on proper and improper weight loss programs

Millions of individuals are involved in weight reduction programs. With the number of undesirable weight loss programs available and a general misconception by many about weight loss, the need for guidelines for proper weight loss programs is apparent.

Based on the existing evidence concerning the effects of weight loss on health status, physiologic processes and body composition parameters, the American College of Sports Medicine makes the following statements and recommendations for weight loss programs.

For the purposes of this position statement, body weight will be represented by two components, fat and fat-free (water, electrolytes, minerals, glycogen stores, muscular tissue, bone, etc.):

1. Prolonged fasting and diet programs that severely restrict caloric intake are scientifically undesirable and can be medically dangerous.

2. Fasting and diet programs that severely restrict caloric intake result in the loss of large amounts of water, electrolytes, minerals, glycogen stores, and other fat-free tissue (including proteins within fat-free tissues), with minimal amounts of fat loss.

3. Mild calorie restriction (500–1000 kcal less than the usual daily intake) results in a smaller loss of water, electrolytes, minerals, and other fat-free tissue, and is less likely to cause malnutrition.

4. Dynamic exercise of large muscles helps to maintain fat-free tissue, including muscle mass and bone density, and results in losses of body weight. Weight loss resulting from an increase in energy expenditure is primarily in the form of fat weight.

5. A nutritionally sound diet resulting in mild calorie restriction coupled with an endurance exercise program along with behavioral modification of existing eating habits is recommended for weight reduction. The rate of sustained weight loss should not exceed 1 kg (2 lb) per week.

6. To maintain proper weight control and optimal body fat levels, a lifetime commitment to proper eating habits and regular physical activity is required.

American College of Sports Medicine position statement on the participation of the female athlete in long-distance running

In the Olympic Games and other international contests, female athletes run distances ranging from 100 meters to 3,000 meters, whereas male athletes run distances ranging from 100 meters through 10,000 meters as well as the marathon (42.2 km). The limitation on distance for women's running events has been defended at times on the grounds that long-distance running may be harmful to the health of girls and women.

Position statement

It is the opinion of the American College of Sports Medicine that females should not be denied the opportunity to compete in long-distance running. There exists no conclusive scientific or medical evidence that long-distance running is contra-indicated for the healthy, trained female athlete. The American College of Sports Medicine recommends that females be allowed to compete at the national and international level in the same distances in which their male counterparts compete.
Source: Med Sci Sports 11 (4) ix–xi 1979

Proposed American College of Sports Medicine position statement on prevention of illness during distance running

Position statement

Based on research findings, it is the position of the American College of Sports Medicine that the following recommendations be employed when conducting distance races or community fun runs. It is ideal to have a medical director who is responsible for the coordination of the preventive and therapeutic aspects related to the fun run and who works closely with the race director.

1. The race organization

(a) Races should be organized to avoid the hottest summer months and the hottest part of the day. Organizers should be very cautious of unseasonable hot days in the early spring, particularly in North America, as entrants will almost certainly not be heat acclimatized.

175

(b) The environmental heat stress on the day should be known and is best measured as WGBT. If WBGT is above 28°C (82°F), the race should be cancelled. If below 28°C, the degrees of heat stress should be conveyed to competitors by the use of color-coded flags at the start of the race to alert them, as follows:

(i) A red flag — high risk: when WBGT is 23–28°C (73–82°F). This signal would indicate that all runners should be aware that heat injury is possible and any person particularly sensitive to heat or humidity should probably not run.

(ii) An amber flag — moderate risk: when WBGT is 18–23°C (65–73°F). It should be remembered that the air temperature and probably also the humidity, and almost certainly the radiant heat at the beginning of the race, will increase during the course of the race if it is conducted in the morning or early afternoon.

(iii) A green flag — low risk: when WBGT is below 18°C(65°F). This in no way guarantees that heat illness will not occur, but indicates only that the risk is low.

(c) All summer events should be scheduled for the early morning, ideally before 9:00 A.M., or in the evening after 6:00 P.M., to minimize solar radiation.

(d) An adequate supply of fluid should be available before the race and every 2–3 km during the race.

(e) Hoses should be available to cool competitors during the race.

(f) Race officials should be educated as to the warning signs of an impending collapse. They should wear an identifiable arm band or badge and be empowered to stop runners who appear to be in difficulty.

(g) Adequate traffic control is necessary.

(h) There should be a ready source of communications from various points on the course to a central organizing point, to meet emergencies.

2. Medical support

(a) Medical organization

Race organizers should alert local hospitals and ambulance services to the event and should take prior arrangements with medical personnel for the care of casualties, especially those suffering from heat injury. The mere fact that an entrant signs a waiver in no way absolves the organizers of the moral and/or legal responsibility.

(b) Medical facilities

(i) These should be available at the race site.

(ii) Staffed with personnel capable of instituting immediate and full-scale resuscitation measures. Apart from the routine resuscitation equipment, ice packs and fans for cooling are required.

(iii) Persons trained in first aid should be stationed along the course with the right to stop runners who exhibit signs of impending heat stroke or other abnormalities.

(iv) One or more ambulances or vans with accompanying medical personnel should follow the competitors at intervals.

(v) Although the emphasis has been on the management of hyperthermia, on cold, wet, and windy days athletes will be cold and require "space blankets," blankets, and warm drinks to prevent hypothermia. Especially vulnerable are the slower athletes who, when lightly clad, will lose heat faster than their rate of metabolic heat production.

3. Competitor education

The education of fun runners has greatly increased in recent years, due largely to the lay person runners' magazines. Distributing sample runners' guidelines at the time of registration, if pre-registration occurs, and also holding clinics before runs are valuable.

The following persons are particularly prone to heat illness: the obese, unfit, dehydrated, those unacclimatized to the heat, the very young and the old, those with a previous history of heat stroke, and anyone who runs while ill. Based on the above information, all competitors should be advised of the following:

(a) Adequate training and fitness are important for full enjoyment of the run and also to prevent heat stroke.

(b) Prior training in the heat will produce heat acclimatization and also reduce the risk of heat injury. It is wise to do as much training as possible at the time of day at which the race will be held.

(c) Fluid consumption before and during the race will also reduce the risk of heat injury, particularly in the longer runs such as the marathon.

(d) Splashing with water or running under available hoses during a race will make runners more comfortable, but is unlikely to reduce the risk of heat injury.

(e) Illness prior to or at the time of the event should preclude competition. This applies to any febrile illness or gastroenteritis.

(f) Competitors should be advised of the early symptoms of heat injury which include excessive sweating, headache, nausea, dizziness, and any gradual impairment of consciousness.

(g) Competitors should be advised to choose a comfortable speed and not to run faster than they have when training.

(h) Competitors are advised to run with a partner, each being responsible for the other's well-being.

Appendix III

Recommended intakes of nutrients

1) Recommended daily intakes (RDI) of energy and nutrients for the UK, 1985 Department of Health and Social Security

Age range years	Occupational category	Energy		Protein
		MJ	Kcal	g
Boys				
9–11		9.5	2280	57
12–14		11.0	2640	66
15–17		12.0	2880	72
Girls				
9–11		8.5	2050	51
12–14		9.0	2150	53
15–17		9.0	2150	53
Men				
18–34	Sedentary	10.5	2510	63
	Moderately active	12.0	2900	72
	Very active	14.0	3350	84
35–64	Sedentary	10.0	2400	60
	Moderately active	11.5	2750	69
	Very active	14.0	3350	84
65–74		10.0	2400	60
75+	sedentary	9.0	2150	54
Women				
18–54	Most occupations	9.0	2150	54
	Very active	10.5	2500	62
55–74		8.0	1900	47
75+	sedentary	7.0	1680	42
Pregnancy		10.0	2400	60
Lactation		11.5	2750	69

Age range years	Occupational category	Thia- min mg	Ribo- flavin mg	Nicotinic acid equiv- alents mg	Ascorbic acid mg	Vitamin A retinol equiv- alents μg	Vitamin D* cholecalci- ferol μg	Cal- cium mg	Iron mg
Boys									
9–11		0.9	1.2	14	25	575	–	700	12
12–14		1.1	1.4	16	25	725	–	700	12
15–17		1.2	1.7	19	30	750	–	600	12
Girls									
9–11		0.8	1.2	14	25	575	–	700	12
12–14		0.9	1.4	16	25	725	–	700	12
15–17		0.9	1.7	19	30	750	–	600	12
Men									
18–34	Sedentary	1.0	1.6	18	30	750	–	500	10
	Moderately active	1.2	1.6	18	30	750	–	500	10
	Very active	1.3	1.6	18	30	750	–	500	10
35–64	Sedentary	1.0	1.6	18	30	750	–	500	10
	Moderately active	1.1	1.6	18	30	750	–	500	10
	Very active	1.3	1.6	18	30	750	–	500	10
65–74	Assuming a	1.0	1.6	18	30	750	–	500	10
75+	sedentary life	0.9	1.6	18	30	750	–	500	10
Women									
18–54	Most occupa- tions	0.9	1.3	15	30	750	–	500	12
	Very active	1.0	1.3	15	30	750	–	500	12
55–74	Assuming a	0.8	1.3	15	30	750	–	500	10
75+	sedentary life	0.7	1.3	15	30	750	–	500	10
Pregnancy		1.0	1.6	18	60	750	10	1200	13
Lactation		1.1	1.8	21	60	1200	10	1200	15

* No dietary sources may be necessary for those exposed to sunlight, but during the winter children and adolescents should receive 10 μ (400 i.u.) daily by supplementation. Adults with inadequate exposure to sunlight, for example those who are housebound, may also need a supplement of 10 μg daily

2) Dietary goals: percentage total energy intake for UK, 1986

Source of energy	Present (%)	Goals (%)
Carbohydrates	40–45	50–55
Fats	40–45	30–35
Proteins	10–12	10–12
Alcohol	6	4

3) Recommended daily dietary allowances (RDAs) for the USA, 1980* (National Academy of Sciences)

	Age (years)	Weight (kg)	(lb)	Height (cm)	(in)	Protein (g)	Vit A (µg RE)	Vit D (µg)	Vit E (mg α-TE)
							Fat-Soluble Vitamins		
Children	7–10	28	62	132	52	34	700	10	7
Males	11–14	45	99	157	62	45	1000	10	8
	15–18	66	145	176	69	56	1000	10	10
	19–22	70	154	177	70	56	1000	7.5	10
	23–50	70	154	178	70	56	1000	5	10
	51+	70	154	178	70	56	1000	5	10
Females	11–14	46	101	157	62	46	800	10	8
	15–18	55	120	163	64	46	800	10	8
	19–22	55	120	163	64	44	800	7.5	8
	23–50	55	120	163	64	44	800	5	8
	51+	55	120	163	64	44	800	5	8
Pregnant						+30	+200	+5	+2
Lactating						+20	+400	+5	+3

	Vit C (mg)	Thiamin (mg)	Riboflavin (mg)	Niacin (mg NE)	Vit B_6 (mg)	Folacin (µg)	Vit B_{12} (µg)
	Water-Soluble Vitamins						
Children	45	1.2	1.4	16	1.6	300	3.0
Males	50	1.4	1.6	18	1.8	400	3.0
	60	1.4	1.7	18	2.0	400	3.0
	60	1.5	1.7	19	2.2	400	3.0
	60	1.4	1.6	18	2.2	400	3.0
Females	60	1.2	1.4	16	2.2	400	3.0
	50	1.1	1.3	15	1.8	400	3.0
	60	1.1	1.3	14	2.0	400	3.0
	60	1.1	1.3	14	2.0	400	3.0
	60	1.0	1.2	13	2.0	400	3.0
	60	1.0	1.2	13	2.0	400	3.0
Pregnant	+20	+0.4	+0.3	+2	+0.6	+400	+1.0
Lactating	+40	+0.5	+0.5	+5	+0.5	+100	+1.0

Minerals	Calcium (mg)	Phosphorus (mg)	Magnesium (mg)	Iron (mg)	Zinc (mg)	Iodine (μg)
Children	800	800	250	10	10	120
Males	1200	1200	350	18	15	150
	1200	1200	400	18	15	150
	800	800	350	10	15	150
	800	800	350	10	15	150
Females	800	800	350	10	15	150
	1200	1200	300	18	15	150
	1200	1200	300	18	15	150
	800	800	300	18	15	150
	800	800	300	18	15	150
	800	700	300	10	15	150
Pregnant	+400	+400	+150		+5	+25
Lactating	+400	+400	+150		+10	+50

	Age (years)	Weight (kg)	Weight (lb)	Height (cm)	Height (in)	Energy needs (with range) (kcal)		Energy needs (with range) (MJ)
Children	7–10	28	62	132	52	2400	(1650–3300)	10.1
Males	11–14	45	99	157	62	2700	(2000–3700)	11.3
	15–18	66	145	176	69	2800	(2100–3900)	11.8
	19–22	70	154	177	70	2900	(2500–3300)	12.2
	23–50	70	154	178	70	2700	(2300–3100)	11.3
	51–75	70	154	178	70	2400	(2000–2800)	10.1
	76+	70	154	178	70	2050	(1650–2450)	8.6
Females	11–14	46	101	157	62	2200	(1500–3000)	9.2
	15–18	55	120	163	64	2100	(1200–3000)	8.8
	19–22	55	120	163	64	2100	(1700–2500)	8.8
	23–50	55	120	163	64	2000	(1600–2400)	8.4
	51–75	55	120	163	64	1800	(1400–2200)	7.6
	76+	55	120	163	64	1600	(1200–2000)	6.7
Pregnancy						+300		
Lactation						+500		

*Please note that these tables (pages 178–181) are currently under revision. Amended tables were unavailable at the time of publication. For additional information and detailed notes please refer to the source document.

4) Dietary goals: percentage total energy intake for USA

Source of energy	Present (%)	Goals (%)
Fat	42	30
Protein	12	12
Carbohydrate	46	58

Glossary

Actin One of the two main contractile proteins found in skeletal muscle cells — the other is myosin

Adaptation The process of change in response to altered stimuli, such as training or diet

Adipocytes The name for cells that store fat as triglyceride

Adipose tissue Tissue consisting of an aggregation of fat cells (adipocytes) containing large reserves of fat — providing both insulation and an energy reserve

ADP (Adenosine diphosphate) The high-energy compound formed when one phosphate group is split from ATP in the process of releasing energy

Aerobic (respiration) Cellular process in which carbohydrate, fat or protein are completely oxidized to CO_2 and water using oxygen

Alcohol An organic compound formed by the fermentation of carbohydrate containing one or more hydroxyl $(-OH)$ groups

Amenorrhoea The complete cessation of normal menstrual function/flow as a result of hormonal changes — often associated with reduced food intakes and low body weights

Amino acid — essential An organic acid containing nitrogen. Large numbers of amino acids combine to form proteins; amino acids termed **essential** must be obtained from the diet because they cannot be synthesised by the body; the basic building block of proteins

Amino acid — limiting In any protein, the amino acid which is furthest below the standard (based on egg protein) is known as the **limiting** amino acid, eg, tryptophon is the limiting amino acid in maize protein; lysine in wheat protein; methionine and cystine in beef protein

Anabolic The synthesis of new material — compounds or tissue — the opposite of catabolic

Anaemia A disease state where lower than normal amounts of haemoglobin in the blood impair oxygen uptake, transportation and utilization

Anaerobic (respiration) Cellular process whereby carbohydrates (mainly glycogen) are incompletely degraded to lactic acid: whilst the total amount of energy liberated is very small, the **rate** is very great

183

Angina   A medical condition whereby the inadequate supply of blood to the contracting muscle of the heart results in severe pain and discomfort

Anorexia   The loss of normal appetite; may develop into the psychological condition known as anorexia nervosa = the complete aversion/rejection of food

ATP (Adenosine triphosphate)   ATP is a nucleotide consisting of a sugar base (adenosine) and three phosphate groups: the chemical bonds between these phosphate groups are known as high-energy bonds and, when broken, energy is released to be used by the various physiological or metabolic processes within the cell requiring energy; thought of as the universal energy currency — the link between the foodstuffs eaten and energy utilization

Bomb calorimetry   The technique used to determine the energy content of materials such as foodstuffs

Buffer   A substance or solution which possesses the capacity to prevent rapid changes in the concentrations of a given ion and pH

Bulimia   The condition where an individual intentionally regurgitates (by self-induced vomiting) the food after it has been eaten — normally if greater than normal amounts of food have been consumed (binges)

Calcium   An essential mineral in the diet; needed in relatively small amounts for the formation of bones and teeth

Calorie   The traditional unit of energy; defined as the heat required to raise 1 g of water from 15 to 16°C; used as a measure of the energy content of food: 1000 calories = 1 kilocalorie

Calorimetry   The measurement of energy expenditure, either directly by the measurement of heat production or indirectly by the measurement of oxygen consumption

Capillary   A tiny thin-walled vessel of small diameter, forming part of a blood vessel network, which aids rapid exchange of substances between the contained fluid and the surrounding tissues, eg oxygen, substrate, end-products, etc

Carbohydrate   A group of complex compounds consisting of carbon, hydrogen and oxygen: one of the main sources of energy in food, eg, sugars and starches. See also Monosaccharide, etc

Carbohydrate-loading   A technique whereby the skeletal muscle glycogen reserves are increased to greater than normal amounts by a combination of exercise and diet

Cardiac output   The rate at which blood is pumped out of the heart; the product of heart rate and stroke volume (the amount of blood pumped per contraction)

Catabolic   The state where tissue or compounds are broken down — the opposite of anabolic

Catalyst   A substance which accelerates a chemical reaction whilst undergoing no permanent change itself, or which may be recovered when the reaction is complete

Chemical compound   A substance composed of two or more elements in definite proportions by weight, irrespective of how the compound is made

Cholesterol   A fat-like substance (a sterol) found in all animal fats and oils; an important component of cell membranes; either present in the diet or synthesized by the body

Chylomicron   A particle of emulsified fat found in the blood following the digestion and absorption of fat

Connective tissue   Material found in many tissues, especially muscle; made up largely from the substance collagen; relatively strong and resistant to stretching, endows strength and structure to tissues such as tendons and ligaments

Coronary heart disease (CHD)   Synonymous with ischaemic heart disease and cardiovascular disease; a group of disease states arising from the failure of the coronary arteries to supply sufficient blood (and oxygen) to the myocardium (heart muscle); most often associated with atherosclerosis (excessive fat deposition) of the vessels providing blood to the heart

Creatine phosphate (CP)   CP may serve as a temporary energetic buffer within the cell to maintain the balance between the rates of energy production and utilization; the high-energy bond may be broken and the energy released used to reform ATP from ADP

Deamination   The process whereby the nitrogen-containing part of amino acids (the amino group) is removed and excreted as urea in the urine

Degradation   The process whereby compounds are broken down

Dietary fibre   The indigestible portion of plant materials such as cellulose, lignin, pectin and gums

Disaccharide   Sugars formed when two monosaccharide molecules combine together, such as sucrose or sugar (glucose and fructose)

Dysmenorroea   The disturbance of normal menstrual function, often temporary

Electrocardiogram (ECG)   A recording of the electrical signals of the heart which can be used to examine cardiac integrity and function

Electrolyte   Dissolved salts or ions in body fluids which carry either a positive or negative electric charge: see also Ion

End-product   The resultant compounds formed by a chemical process, eg CO_2, water, ammonia

Energy   The capacity to perform work

Energy crisis (deficit)   A condition where the rate of energy resynthesis cannot keep pace with the rate of energy utilization, resulting in a reduction, and deficit, in

185

the availability of energy to support physiological and metabolic processes.

Enzyme Complex protein molecules that act as biological catalysts (ie, increase the rate of a chemical reaction without itself being changed at the end of the reaction). Normally enzymes are highly specific to the substrates with which they react. The relative activity of an enzyme is normally controlled by a variety of other chemical compounds known as cofactors and can be increased or decreased very rapidly

Ergogenic aids From the Greek 'ergon' meaning work, ergogenic aids theoretically endow the user with an increased capacity to perform muscular work

Exercise intensity (relative) The degree of physiological and metabolic stress imposed on an individual during muscular exercise is related to the severity of the exercise task. Normally, exercise intensity is related to the maximum aerobic capacity of an individual, eg, 60–80% $\dot{V}O_2$max

Fasciculus A small bundle of skeletal muscle fibres

Fatigue See Energy Crisis

Fats The group of complex organic compounds for chemical substances including triglycerides, phospholipids and sterols; more correctly known as lipids

Fatty acids Together with glycerol, fatty acids form triglycerides. When triglycerides are broken down, fatty acids are released. Three classes of fatty acids are described according to the number of double bonds between the carbon atoms: saturated: none, unsaturated: one, polyunsaturated: two or more. Polyunsaturated fatty acids include the essential fatty acids (linoleic and linolenic acids) that have to be provided in the diet

FG fibres Fast glycolytic skeletal muscle fibres: fast contracting, fast fatiguing, with a high capacity to utilize glycogen anaerobically; often referred to as Type IIb or white fibres

Fluid compartment Body water is contained within different regions of the cells: intracellular — the space within the cells, extracellular — outside the plasma membranes of the cells

FOG fibres Fast oxidative glycolytic skeletal muscle fibres: the intermediate sub-group between the more oxidative SO fibres and the more glycolytic FG fibres; can only be converted to FG fibres; often referred to as Type IIa fibres

Fructose The monosaccharide found in all sweet fruits; combines with glucose to make sucrose; also known as levulose

Fuel The chemical substance from which energy is derived, eg carbohydrate and fat

Galactose A monosaccharide resembling glucose in most of its properties but is less soluble and less sweet; combined with glucose makes lactose — the principal carbohydrate in milk

Gluconeogenesis   The formation of carbohydrates from molecules which are not themselves carbohydrate, such as protein and fat, eg, the synthesis of glucose from amino acids, lactate, alanine and glycerol primarily by the liver (and kidney)

Glucose   The most frequently occurring monosaccharide in the diet

Glucosyl unit   The carbohydrate molecule resulting from the degradation of glycogen in glycogenolysis

Glycerol   A component of triglycerides along with fatty acids; a sugar alcohol

Glycogen   The storage form of glucose in animal cells, mainly liver and skeletal muscle; a polysaccharide which is the primary carbohydrate storage form in animals

Glycogenolysis   The specific degradation of glycogen into smaller compounds

Glycolysis   The degradation of carbohydrate, both as glucose or glycogen, into smaller compounds which then may either enter the mitochondria for oxidation or be converted to lactate

Haem-Iron   Iron of animal origin, normally associated with protein (eg, haemoglobin); preferentially absorbed in the gut over mineral salts of iron

Haemoglobin   The iron-containing protein in red blood cells responsible for the transportation of oxygen from the lungs to the cells of the body via the blood stream

Homeostasis   The maintenance of a physiological or metabolic equilibrium within the body; a constant internal environment

Hydration   The restitution of normal fluid reserves of the body

Hydrolysis   The splitting of a chemical bond between elements in a compound using water

Hyper/hypoglycaemia   Hyper: greater than normal levels of glucose in the blood; hypo: Lower than normal levels of glucose in the blood

Hyper/hypothermia   Hyper: greater than normal body temperture; hypo: lower than normal body temperature

Hyper/hypotonic   Hyper: having an osmotic pressure greater than that of the solution to which it is compared — in this context, normally body fluids; Hypo: having an osmotic pressure lower than that of the solution to which it is compared — in this context, normally body fluids: See also: **osmosis**

Hyponutrition   The condition where the intake of food is so low that the nutrient intake is insufficient to satisfy the body's requirements

Ileum   The posterior or latter part of the small intestine (ie, precedes the colon or large intestine)

Intermediate   In this context, a compound formed by the degradation of a storage compound: glycolytic intermediates are the compounds formed as glycogen is converted to pyruvate (eg, glucose-6-phospate)

Interstitial   The space between cells

Intestine   The part of the alimentary canal leading from the stomach to the anus

Ion   A single atom or group of atoms that have gained or lost one or more electrons and so has an electric charge. Cations are formed when electrons are lost (eg, Na^+); anions when gaining an electron (eg, Cl^-)

Isokinetic   Pertaining to the generation of muscular force which will vary over the range of joint angle, eg a typical extension

Isometric   Pertaining to the generation of muscular force without discernable shortening of muscle length, eg a static contraction

Isotonic   Pertaining to a state of equal tension or activity; muscle: equal tension throughout the range of motion; solutions: equal osmotic pressure between two solutions

Jejunum   The middle part of the small intestine between the duodenum and the ileum; primary region of food absorption

Joule   The SI unit of energy, work or heat: 4.184 joules = 1 calorie

Ketone (bodies)   Intermediate products of fat metabolism produced when fatty acids release exceeds utilization; can be used by muscle during exercise as an energy source and by the brain

Kilocalorie   The most commonly used unit of energy: 1 kcal = 1000 calories = 4.184 joules

Kilojoule   The SI unit of energy, work or heat: 1 kJ = 1000 joules, 4.184 kJ = 1 kcal

Krebs cycle   The series of reactions catalysed by enzymes in the mitochondria whereby pyruvate and other intermediates are oxidized to CO_2 and water generating ATP

Lactate/lactic acid   Lactic acid is the anaerobic product of glycolysis formed when the rate of pyruvate production exceeds pyruvate oxidation; under physiological conditions, this rapidly dissociates to lactate$^-$ and hydrogen$^+$ ions

Lactose   The disaccharide primarily found in milk, glucose and galactose

Limiting   That which constrains or restricts a given quality or extent of a physiological/metabolic process

Lipoprotein   A combination of lipid and protein formed by the liver as a means of specifically transporting fats in plasma to target tissues

Lymphatic system   A system of vessels pervading the body in which lymph (a blood plasma-like substance) circulates — also connects with the venous circulation

Macromineral   Minerals required by the body in relatively large quantities, eg calcium, iron

Maltose   The disaccharide formed by combining two glucose molecules; normally found in plant material

188

Manganese   An essential mineral

Megajoule   A unit of energy, heat or work: 1 MJ = 1000 kJ = 240 kcal

Metabolic fate   Ultimate end product of metabolism

Metabolism   The sum of all chemical processes/reactions taking place in the body or organs or cells. Primarily involves the breaking down of complex organic chemicals to simpler molecules

Metabolite   Intermediate in metabolism

Metabolize   To break down complex organic molecules to simpler molecules

Mineral   A naturally occurring substance produced by inorganic processes; ie. not of plant or animal origin

Mitochondria (singular: **mitochondrion**)   Specialized structure within cells with specific capability to oxidize substrates, releasing energy bound as ATP

Molecule   The smallest group of atoms bound together as either an element or compound which has a free existence

Monosaccharide   The basic buidling block of carbohydrates; a simple sugar with the general formula $C_nH_{2n}O_n$ where n usually ranges from 3–7: glucose is a 6 carbon monosaccharide — two or more monosaccharides join to form disaccharides or polysaccharides

Myosin   One of the two main proteins of contraction found in skeletal muscle cells, the other is actin

Nicotinic acid — Niacin — Nicotinamide   Vitamin B_3 — one of the B complex vitamins: important component of coenzymes, required for the oxidation of carbohydrate and fat

Nutrient   A substance conveying, serving as, or providing nourishment, eg, carbohydrate

Osmosis   Diffusion of a solvent (eg, water) through a semi-permeable membrane from a less concentrated to a more concentrated solution, tending to equalize the concentrations on both sides of the membrane

Osmolality   The osmotic potential of a solution

Osteoporosis   A medical condition where the demineralization of bone causes a degeneration of the bone matrix resulting in weakness and fragility

Oxidation   The addition of oxygen to a compound; primarily takes place within the mitochondria where substrates are fully combusted in the presence of oxygen to CO_2, water and energy

Peptide   Substances resulting from the breakdown of proteins where two or more amino acids are joined together

Performance   In sporting terms, the capacity to perform work in relation to that specific sporting activity, eg, time, distance, height, speed, etc

Photosynthesis The process by which the cells of green plants synthesize complex organic substances (such as carbohydrates, fats and proteins) from simple inorganic materials (eg, CO_2, water and nitrogen) using the energy of light, with the liberation of O_2

Physiological Relating to the functions of an animal or man as a living organism; the processes essential to maintain life, eg, breathing, digestion, excretion, etc

Polysaccharide A carbohydrate which when hydrolysed yields ten or more monosaccharides (eg, starch)

Potassium A very reactive alkali metal which as a mineral salt is an essential component of the diet

Protein A complex molecule composed of amino acids joined together by peptide linkages: essential constituents of the living cell and must be provided in the diet to make good tissue wastage and accommodate growth

Pyruvate (pyruvic acid) An important intermediary compound in energy metabolism. It can be formed by the degradation of many substrates (eg, glycogen, glucose, some amino acids, etc) and can be converted to lactic acid, transaminated to alanine, converted back to glycogen or oxidized by the Krebs cycle.

Recruitment The process by which skeletal muscle fibres are stimulated to contract and participate in the generation of force.

Respiratory quotient (RQ) Determined from the relative rates of oxygen uptake and carbon dioxide production; can be used as a general indicator of relative substrate oxidation either at rest or during moderate exercise; also referred to as respiratory exchange ratio

Resting or basal metabolic rate The energy expended by the body at rest sufficient to support the metabolic processes necessary for life, eg protein turnover, ventilation, circulation, etc; measured under specific conditions.
BMR — basal metabolic rate

Risk factors A collection of different lifestyle characteristics and metabolic characteristics which have been shown statistically to increase the probability of contracting a specific disease, eg coronary heart disease

Sodium A very reactive alkali metal which as a mineral salt is an essential component of the diet

SO fibres Slow oxidative skeletal muscle fibres: slow contracting, slow fatiguing, with a high capacity to utilize substrates (particularly fats) oxidatively; often referred to as Type I or red fibres

Starch The storage form/compound of glucose in plant cells — a polysaccharide

Steady-state A dynamic condition whereby the physiological and metabolic processes have fully adjusted to meet the demands of an altered state (eg exercise); in this condition, the processes have stabilized or plateaued out at a new level

Stroke volume The volume of blood discharged from the ventricles of the heart per contraction or heart beat

Submaximal exercise An exercise task where the relative exercise intensity is less than the $\dot{V}O_2$ max of the given individual (eg, endurance exercise)

Substrate A chemical substance or compound which is changed in an enzyme-controlled reaction to a different compound (product); usually refers to fuels used to provide energy

Sucrose Common household 'sugar': a disaccharide of glucose and fructose

Supramaximal exercise An exercise task where the relative exercise intensity is greater than an individual's $\dot{V}O_2$max (eg, sprinting)

Synthesis The formation of a new product from other compounds or substances by a single or multi-stepped enzyme-controlled reaction

Taper To reduce slowly. Normally used in terms of reducing the volume of training prior to competition

Thermic effect of feeding (TEF) The increase in metabolic rate observed after the consumption of food

Thermogenesis The production of heat by metabolic processes, normally by the splitting of chemical bonds, eg, the synthesis and utilization of ATP

Trace element Those elements essential to the body but only needed in very small amounts (eg several milligrams a day or less)

Triglyceride One of the many different types of fat formed by the union of glycerol and fatty acids; the principle storage form of fat in the body; also referred to as triacylglycerol

Turnover The form given to the collective process of synthesis and degradation of a compound or group of compounds, eg, the continual process whereby proteins are formed from amino acids and then broken down again in the body

Twitch A single contraction induced by the electrical stimulation of skeletal muscle fibre(s)

Ventilation The process by which air is taken into the lungs and then expelled by movements of the intercostal muscles and diaphragm

$\dot{V}O_2$ Term given to denote the rate at which oxygen is taken up by the body; usually expressed in litres per minute or millilitres per kg body weight per minute (mls/kg/min)

$\dot{V}O_2$max The maximal rate of oxygen uptake for an individual; reflects the greatest rate of oxidative processes; often referred to as the maximal oxidative capacity or aerobic capacity of an individual

Index

In this index, bold page numbers refer to entries in the Glossary.

Index